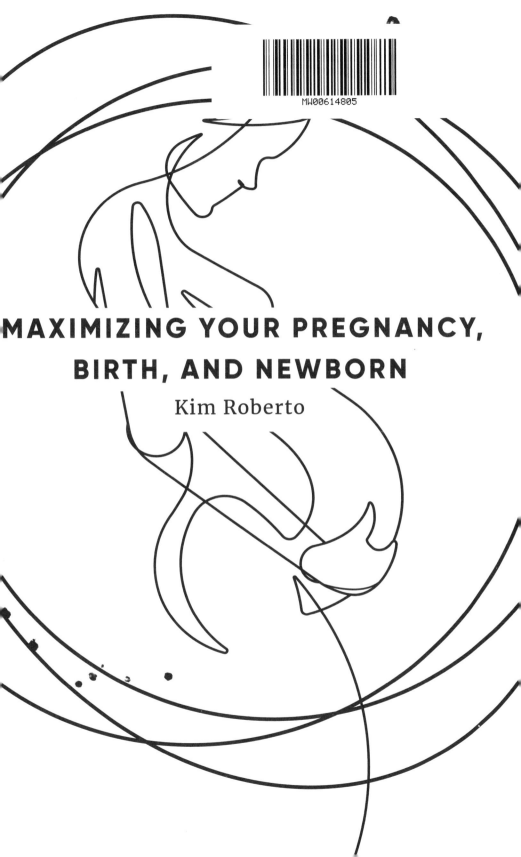

MAXIMIZING YOUR PREGNANCY, BIRTH, AND NEWBORN

Kim Roberto

Disclaimer
The information contained in this book is provided for educational purposes only. It is not a substitute for the advice provided by your physician or other healthcare professionals. Kimberly Roberto is not a medical doctor, and the information in this book should not be used to diagnose or treat a health problem or disease.

Always consult your Holistic Primary Healthcare Professional before adjusting, adding to, or stopping any diet, supplements, exercise, or medical regimen.

The information in this book should not be considered complete, or used as a course of treatment for a particular individual. It should not be used in place of a visit with, call to, consultation with, or advice of your physician or other qualified healthcare provider. Information obtained in this book is not exhaustive and does not cover all diseases, conditions, procedures, or treatments. You should never disregard medical advice or delay seeking treatment due to information you have read in this book.

The contents of this book are based upon the opinions of the author. The author and publisher make no representations or warranties as to the accuracy or completeness of the contents of this book. The authors and publisher disclaim any liability arising directly or indirectly from the use of this book and are not liable for any misuse of the material contained in this book. Any references to citations, quotes, or any other third-party material is for informational purposes only and should be verified by the reader and their medical professional. Maximized Living has not verified any third-party materials included in this book and makes no warranty or guarantees either express or implied.

ISBN 9781933936000

51499 >

9 781933 936000

Table of Contents

Recipes

Congratulations!

I am so excited for you and the expectations ahead with a growing family. It is an amazing time in your life and I wish to encourage you through the knowledge and wisdom this book shares along this spectacular journey. The purpose of this book is to provide accurate information, discuss what to expect, and describe what is happening with your body and your growing baby. Further, this book works to outline your options for prenatal care, the birth process, and what lies beyond. Please know if you have questions or concerns along the way, I welcome you to contact either Dr. Fred Roberto or myself for assistance or feedback (see Contact section). Historically in our practice, mothers and babies consistently exposed to MaxLiving's "5 Essentials®"–which are comprised of Core Chiropractic, Nutrition, Mindset, Oxygen & Exercise, and Mimimize Toxins–experience far more pleasant pregnancies, easier births, fewer complications, and most importantly, a head start on a lifetime of good health.

It is important to understand the birth process is a natural, beautiful progression set in place since the beginning of time. It is not a disease or condition requiring "treatment." Your body was equipped for this since you yourself were in the womb, and can accomplish exactly what it needs to throughout the pregnancy process. Have faith in your body, the miracle of childbirth, and place full trust in your Creator.

Remember, you always have choices. It is your body, your baby, but also, your responsibility to thoroughly research the pros and cons of all available options. In this book, I do my best to share basic information. However, it is still up to you to conduct any further research.

****

Introduction - My Birth Stories

After Fred and I were married, we were very excited to start a family. He was a newly licensed Chiropractor with a focus on pregnancy and pediatrics, and I was only 24, working full time for General Electric. When the subject of children was broached, Fred would inadvertently discuss things like (gasp!) natural birth and avoiding vaccines, topics so unfamiliar to me. I would scoff with indignation, thinking, "What in the world is he even talking about?! Of course I will have an epidural! Of course our babies will be vaccinated!"

Being the brilliant man he is and knowing me well, he carried out the perfect plan by gently opening my mind to a naturally healing world I was never exposed to previously. Fred wisely played off my voracious appetite for learning through my love of reading by merely leaving a pile of books on the table.

As a result of my desire to poke holes through his entire stance on the matter, and to put a quick end to these silly discussions, begrudgingly, I picked up the book at the top of the stack. The title was "Vaccines: Are They Really Safe and Effective?" by Neil Z. Miller. By the time I reached Chapter Two, page 4, I was forever converted. I decided right then and there–absolutely no vaccines for our future precious babies! Also, coming quickly to the realization that if I was so wrong about vaccines, I knew I'd best look into this "natural childbirth" thing too.

It is important to note this book is not anti-vaccination, instead, it is about pro-education and informed parental consent. We recognize our choice may not be right for everyone, however, if you have not yet delved into the very real and controversial vaccine issue, I would encourage you to make this a top learning priority. Otherwise, you may possibly be forced to make a life altering and hasty decision–most likely under extreme pressure. There is a plethora of pro-vaccine information out there but unbiased and clear information is much more difficult to locate unless you know where to look. This book provides credible facts and statistics to help round out your research so you are able to make more fully informed decisions.

Now that I had become a reading and research machine on this topic, would sit my husband down and bombard him with all I had learned. Spouting with disbelief I would commentate, "Can you believe this?! Wait! Listen to THIS one!" Fred would politely nod his head, raise his eyebrows, allowing me to bask in my full glory of these new profound revelations. The entire time he was relishing the fact that another mind had been opened–as this way of life WAS his way life! The plan he had so strategically laid in front of me like a little egg hatched open like a baby spring chicken, and I was now more than ready to cross that road to get to the other side.

We decided to enroll in natural childbirth classes called the "Bradley Method," never looking back once we became pregnant. Many of Fred's colleagues were opting for home births to avoid potential medical interventions and the cold, unfriendly clinical nature of a hospital. Although fully committed to natural birth, I was unable to wrap my head around actually delivering a baby at home, on our bed, or, in a child's blow up pool smack dab in the middle of our living room. At the time, it seemed to be too risky, but reflecting back, it now sounds like it could have been a beautiful and glorious experience. Unfortunately, it was an obstacle I was not able to overcome. So, combined with my sometimes admittedly rebellious, "You can't tell me what I can or can't do!" attitude, I was confident I could birth our baby at a hospital on my own terms. Fred, however, would always say, "I'll do whatever you want, just know though, we are entering the lion's den when we walk into that hospital." I have a tendency to be a bit too big for my britches at times and thought to myself, "Bring it on, lions….just bring it on!"

In 1997 I gave birth to our first son, James, 100% naturally and on our own terms. However, it seems only fitting I share how we arrived there and disclose the rest of the story.

As I had gained 50 pounds during the pregnancy, experiencing considerable swelling, the midwife instructed I must be on bed rest with three weeks still to go until my due date. Thankfully my water broke two short days later, which took place before my first contraction. This was somewhat troublesome as typically, when the water breaks prior to labor, modern medicine inevitably wants to intervene. Despite this, we decided to wait until my contractions were closer together before going to the hospital. Labor progressed as usual and while we waited, I am certain we looked like super ninjas, swatting away the continual offers of drugs, epidurals, ultrasounds, stripping of membranes, and other potentially scary interventions buzzing around our heads. We were feeling pretty good at the time and confident about things.

One thing though in looking back, I wish to have known then what I know now regarding nutrition. With every contraction, I was vomiting, as prior to labor I decided to consume a giant spaghetti dinner at a local restaurant—what I thought at the time was a fantastic idea in protest of my seemingly unfair sentence banishing me to bed rest.

Eventually, my cervix dilated to 10 cm. and I received the go-ahead to push, so push I did. I pushed for 5 hours! During labor, a wonderful midwife was on call, entirely supportive and on board with our birth plan. Unfortunately, there was this thing called a shift change and the sweet angel floated away—and a not so nice, very impatient doctor roared in….just like the "lions" Fred had warned me about. He definitely was not accommodating as the midwife, and quite a rude awakening to our birthing process.

To make things worse, he recommended Pitocin, which is a drug meant to unnaturally speed the delivery along and can make labor contractions far more severe and painful. He immediately started urging a C-section be performed, his scare tactics raging in full force. He said terribly horrifying things to a first-time expectant mother such as "Your baby is stuck in the birth canal!", "Your baby can't breathe" and, "Your baby could die!"

But Fred and I stayed strong.

Ok, I lied. Only Fred stayed strong. I was crumpled in pain, overwhelmed with doubt. We continued to stay committed to the natural birth process when the doctor turned to me and asked, "Why, am I even here?!" I was not in any state to respond, but had the wherewithal to notice my husband coming in fast with his fist clenched, knowing Fred was perfectly capable of knocking the pompous doctor out in one shot. I was also (pretty) sure my husband wouldn't actually "hit" him, but really was not up to the adventure of finding out. Thankfully, my mother, seeing my distress, spontaneously erupted into a hysterical outburst, screaming, stomping her feet and storming out of the room. We were relieved when the doctor followed suit. Fred dropped his clenched fist and swooped to my side so we could regroup.

The nurses were also angels sent from heaven above. I continued to push until they saw a baby's head crowning. This should have been great news, but not exactly, as this little person had shoulders, and I knew what that meant. Shoulders are wider than a head, and I quit–announcing I was done, please put it back–I want to go home. My husband went into pep talk mode, and the brilliant nurse-angel ran for oxygen, gave Fred a knowing look, and placed the mask on my face. I suddenly felt like a new person, full of vigor, ready to get this job done! With a quarter of a push, our perfect son James Anthony–8 pounds, 6 oz.–entered this world, and we were forever changed.

The nurses were amazed I had not torn during delivery, as I had refused an episiotomy–even with those big shoulders of his! Months previous to this moment I used a technique called Perineal Massage (see appendix) to naturally stretch the vaginal area using specific massage techniques to avoid tearing during childbirth. Within 30 minutes I was up walking around, so ecstatic I had accomplished this marvelous feat called giving birth! The joy of bringing a new life into the world to this day is still unsurpassed.

Soon after James Anthony's birth, we had two more children, between 1997 and 2000. They were also hospital births, 100% non-medicated, and on our terms. Their births were much less dramatic, and nurses and staff were amazed by how smooth these "natural births" were! These were not itty bitty babies and again, I was thankful not to tear with either of them regardless of long labor times.

The hospital released us each time within 24 hours. Our children thrived, and so did I.

As I mentioned previously, looking back, wish I would have chosen home births. Things are very different now and people are encouraged to stay out of the hospital if at all possible. There is much risk of unintentionally veering away from your desired birth plan, succumbing to fear under tremendous pressure, potentially experiencing shaming, and undergoing unnecessary procedures. You may experience un-due scrutiny from complete strangers regarding your decisions, including the risk of child services being contacted if someone "believes" you are not serving your baby's best interest due to their own lack of knowledge.

For over twenty years I have been fortunate enough to assist parents through healthy pregnancies and births, continuing to help raise them into healthy children and then on to young adults, finding I still desire to do so much more. This book is a result of that desire, created just for you, who just like me, are searching for truth.

I hope this book provides you the information to inspire the desire to seek more knowledge, to learn, and to embrace the miracle of childbirth and encourages you to contemplate and research each childbirth decision on your own.

Many Blessings,
Kimberly Roberto & Dr. Fred Roberto

CHAPTER 1
Prenatal Considerations

The Gift

The progression of conception is glorious and nothing short of awe-inspiring. Think of the marvel of one egg from a woman, and a single sperm from a man uniting together to intentionally yet spontaneously create life. Remarkably, 2 cells become 4, dividing into 16, over and over again until eventually achieving a phenomenal count of approximately 74 trillion cells. This division, replication, and growth transpires all in a matter of 9 short months!

Let's look at the miraculous progression of this priceless life forming within the womb. Upon comprehending the deliberate development which takes place, it reveals this is quite clearly more than "just a blob of cells." The first part to develop is the Central Nervous System (CNS) and this is no coincidence as it consists of the brain, spinal cord, and nerves. After all, the Central Nervous System (CNS) controls every cell, tissue, and organ in your body, which I will discuss in more detail later.

Next, the heart and lungs develop, followed by eyelids, ear canals, fingers, toes, bones, genitals, major organs, and muscles. Eventually, tiny buds for teeth, eyelashes, eyebrows, fingernails, hair, and one of a kind fingerprints develop. Your baby starts to move around, hear your voice, taste sweet and sour, and is able to open and close their eyes. All of this amazing metamorphosis takes place in the comfort of mom's womb.

It is imperative to understand a baby is very vulnerable to outside influences while developing. Babies can potentially be subjected to things which do not support this extraordinary evolving process, possibly affecting healthy development. For instance, the quality (organic vs. non-organic) and type of food the mother consumes is crucial. Turn to fruits, veggies, free-range eggs, and grass-fed beef rather than processed, pre-packaged foods. The toxins an expectant mother is exposed to every day, whether through drinking water, toothpaste, pesticides, plastics, or skin lotions, may silently impact this little life. Also, any medical interventions administered and various stress levels encountered can negatively affect development. We live in a time where there is considerably more toxic exposure than ever. The levels of processed food, significantly less physical activity, and high stress from the hectic lives we bring on ourselves have rarely been experienced previously.

Pregnancy and birth are topics which could easily fill an additional four books, but it is important to start here in terms of understanding the human body and principals of true good health. In the United States of America, we approach pregnancy as a "medical condition" which must be "treated" as opposed to a completely natural process to be embraced, supported, and respected.

What I am about to say is not meant to offend anyone or come across as judgmental. There are of course situations when emergency or modern medical technology is required, and thankful we have access to it in this great country! However, during pregnancy, unnecessary procedures are consistently insisted upon and performed due to "standard and customary reasons," or, for "ease and convenience," regrettably at times to accommodate the doctor's schedule, or for the purpose of monetary gain.

Sadly, women have innocently handed over their natural rights endowed by their Creator when bringing new life into the world. Instead, they succumb to the tidal wave of convention and procedure. Women are "told" what their due dates are and how much weight they should gain. They are subjected to numerous tests, expected to undergo many medical interventions such as inductions, stripping of membranes, epidurals, C-sections, and episiotomies. In addition, sensitive body systems are exposed to toxic synthetic pharmaceuticals for pain. Expectant mothers are often told to forgo breastfeeding, instead encouraged to reach for the ease of a bottle of man-made formula. Ironically, formula is designed to be as close to breast milk as possible, so why not just recommend breast milk?

It is important to decide how you want to proceed with your prenatal period and delivery as soon as possible. There are many options available, so I encourage you to consider them all to make an educated decision on what you feel is best for your family.

These decisions are not something to be taken lightly, and I wish to inspire you to seek knowledge in order to develop a stronger connection between

Before You Become Pregnant

As with any significant endeavor in life, it is always advisable to do your research. When one purchases a home or a vehicle, there is much exploration and preparation prior to ensure a positive long-term outcome.

It is no different when considering having a family. Prior to pregnancy, it is advised to schedule a wellness check with your primary Holistic Health Care Provider to determine at that time if one is healthy enough to handle a pregnancy. This allows you to wisely prepare, ensuring your body is ready to provide a physiologically healthy environment for your baby to thrive and grow in.

If you are planning to become pregnant within the next year, I encourage you to track your ovulation cycle through methods suggested by "The Couple to Couple League" natural family planning, or the "Marquette Method," a store-purchased fertility monitor (see appendix) to best predict your ovulation times.

In the book's opening section, I mentioned MaxLiving's "5 Essentials" which are comprised of "Core Chiropractic, Nutrition, Mindset, Oxygen & Exercise, and Minimizing Toxins." Incorporated are some suggestions for each segment to help you prepare for your upcoming pregnancy.

Core Chiropractic - Spine & Nervous System

Consider first having your spine and nervous system evaluated. The nervous system controls every single organ, tissue, and process in your body. This includes blood flow to your uterus, ovulation, and hormonal regulation. Signal interference to your nervous system at any level may compromise how your body functions. It is also critical your pelvis be in alignment. This can help ensure proper positioning of the baby and allow for proper stretching of the ligaments.

A MaxLiving Chiropractor will be able to properly address any misalignments and nerve interference before you become pregnant.

Mindset

It is critical to work through past traumas and hurts you may have experienced. Emotional turmoil not only interferes with the ability to become pregnant, but can lead to a stressful pregnancy, including postpartum depression after your baby is born. Work to identify any underlying issues where forgiveness might be in order, or traumas, injustices, and stress that may be affecting your life. This is also important for preventing disease and for your overall health.

Stress has tangible physiological effects that could interfere with fertility, conception and a healthy pregnancy. These effects include changes in mood, immune system suppression, elevated blood pressure, sleep problems, hormone dysregulation, and more! [1]

Here are a few strategies to assist you in working through any emotional issues:

- Talk through things with people you trust and who listen well
- Therapy
- Engage in positive self-talk and repeated affirmations
- Meditation and/or spiritual practices

The healing process is different for everyone and is a journey that may not have easy answers, but the more you move towards healing, the more peace you will experience.

Evaluate the amount of stress in your life and look for ways to reduce it. For example, if you have a stressful job, consider a different company, or figure out creative ways to work less hours or work from home. If your relationships are strained, seek help from trusted friends, mentors, or professional counselors. If you have other children, begin to make a plan for what happens when your new baby enters the family dynamics.

Nutrition

Wise planning in this area is strongly advised prior to becoming pregnant. For example, it is imperative to ensure that those vital B vitamins and various minerals are not deficient. If you are deficient, your baby will also most likely be deficient, BUT their deficiency would woefully occur during crucial times of development, potentially impacting them–and you–for the rest of their life.

For example, the mere mention of the serious birth defect Spina Bifida is well known to send chills of terror through expectant parents. This potentially crippling disorder can simply be a result of the mother not possessing enough of the essential B vitamin (Folate/Folic Acid) during those first crucial weeks of pregnancy.[2] So, how much better to know these deficiencies ahead of time and address and manage them prior to pregnancy, rather than discovering too late and potentially impacting the child and family's quality of life for years to come.

It is important to provide your body the essential nutrients it needs, especially as you prepare to conceive a child. The sooner you start implementing nutritional changes, the healthier and easier it will be while you are pregnant and beyond. See the nutrition section of this book or the MaxLiving "Align Your Health" book for more detailed information.

One area really not up for debate is how crucial it is to wean–or stop cold turkey–tobacco products and alcohol. None of these are conducive to conception or to pregnancy. Although there is controversy whether or not caffeine can affect your baby while in utero or nursing, it is never a bad idea to cut back, especially if you feel "addicted" or suffer from negative side effects when you go without.

Throughout this book you will frequently see the reminder to stay hydrated. Most people walk around in a chronic state of dehydration without even realizing it. A good rule of thumb is to take your weight and divide it by 2. This is the recommended amount of water in ounces to drink every day. For example, if you weigh 130 lbs, you would drink 65 ounces of water per day. Of course that number should go up if you are exercising, but is a general guideline. This will be a good habit to get into since your hydration needs will greatly increase with pregnancy and nursing.

Nutraceuticals

Of course, it is ideal to get the nutrients you need from the food you eat. However, there are several nutraceuticals most women need. As mentioned earlier, is advisable to have nutritional testing done to identify potential deficiencies. Visit your MaxLiving Doctor for more information on nutritional testing and to ensure there are no contraindicative issues with medications you may have been previously prescribed for.

Prenatal Multivitamin – It is important a prenatal vitamin be natural, free of toxins, bio-available (easily absorbed, assimilated and used by the body), and effective.

Essential Fatty Acids– Good, quality fats are lacking in the Standard American Diet, but many supplements may come from less than desirable sources and not actually containing what is stated on the bottle.

Bone Strengthening Nutraceutical – Strong bones are essential before, during, and after pregnancy. Bone supporting nutraceuticals contain nutrients that can help enhance bone strength for a healthy foundation.

Recommendation: MaxLiving Prenatal Daily Essentials Packets! These comprehensive packets combine all three of these into a convenient, easy-to-use packet.

Oxygen and Exercise

If you are not already, this is the perfect time to get in the habit of exercising, as it is not ideal to start an exercise program once you are already pregnant. Implementing exercise in your daily regiment long before you conceive allows you to build up your strength and endurance, before continuing to work out during your pregnancy. It is widely known and accepted that exercising and moving your body during pregnancy leads to an easier pregnancy, smoother labor/delivery, and quicker recovery times. Music to the ears of any expectant mother. If you are not interested, or unable to exercise, please consider simply moving your body. Walk, jog, dance, play a sport, hike–whatever makes you happy and gets your body moving.

Minimize Toxins

Detoxing Your Body

While detoxification is extremely important to a healthy body, it is imperative you not do any type of detoxification program while you are pregnant or nursing, as you may be releasing toxins into your body that may negatively affect your baby. If you suspect you have a considerable toxic load, it is a great idea to go through a detoxification program PRIOR to pregnancy.

The typical culprits are toxins such as mold, heavy metals (aluminum, mercury, and lead), and many other environmental toxins. Some of these are difficult to identify and even more difficult to detoxify, so I encourage you to work with a healthcare provider who is well educated and experienced on these processes.

This would also be the time to remove any amalgam (silver) fillings as they contain mercury. This will ensure there is no continued exposure. It is imperative you seek out a biological dentist who follows a safe protocol for removing amalgam fillings. Never remove or add amalgam fillings while you are pregnant or nursing.

Speaking of teeth, you should also be checked for any possible infections from previous root canals, etc., and for any type of periodontal disease. There have been studies linking periodontal disease to things like premature births and low birth weights.[3]

Perspiring–or sweating–is also a terrific way to detoxify. Using an infrared sauna can also be useful to help detoxify your body.

Epsom salt baths are wonderful, and I suggest taking them frequently. Not only are they detoxifying, but they are also relaxing and allow you to decompress. Simply fill a bathtub with water and add 1-2 cups of Epsom salts. You can even add 1-2 cups of baking soda and 1-2 cups of hydrogen peroxide to further the detoxification. After everything has dissolved, add 2-8 drops of your favorite essential oil for additional therapeutic and relaxing effects.

Detoxing Your Home

The EPA now estimates our indoor environments are even more toxic than the outdoor air we breathe.[4] We are exposed to numerous toxins in our own homes by cleaning products, personal care products, chemicals used in building materials, furniture, fabrics, the contents in our medicine cabinets, and, even, the food in our refrigerators and pantries.

Making the switch from toxic products to non-toxic is often an easy one. There are toxin-free versions of just about everything you can think of. You will also want to become well-educated on what you will be using for your baby and what your baby will be exposed to in your home. You can talk to your MaxLiving doctor for more information specific to your area or use these valuable resources to help you along the way.

By moving your mindset and lifestyle habits up to a healthier level, you place yourself in the best position for conception as well as a healthy happy pregnancy, birth process, and parenthood.

****

CHAPTER 2
Nutrition During Pregnancy

Keep in mind you will be eating for two now and everything you put in your mouth and on your body is shared with your growing baby. The ideal nutrition plan is always important, but especially vital during pregnancy. This means whole-food based and as close to the original source as possible, naturally raised and/or cultivated. Embrace this time in your life to step up your commitment to a solid, sustainable nutrition plan you can carry well beyond your pregnancy. This also helps establish success for your growing family in terms of their long-term health.

Unfortunately, the original typical "S.A.D."–Standard American Diet–we know now has done great damage to several generations of our population. The first food pyramid was created by the Swedish National Board of Health and Welfare in 1972.[5] The creator was discovered to have ulterior motives benefiting from a retail market. The USDA then in turn created our own food pyramid in 1992, updated it in 2005, and transformed it again to "MyPlate" in 2011. This transformation was a complete do-over and whoopsidaisy, recognizing significant negative consequences to the public in their efforts over decades to push and promote an unhealthy amount of grains in the RDA, or Recommended Daily Allowances.[6]

This is evidenced by skyrocketing statistics of heart disease, diabetes, prostate cancer, breast cancer, and obesity–the five chronic diseases North Americans are most likely to die from. If you look back as little as 100 years ago, these problems did not even exist. What went so wrong and when? It is a complex question which provides various answers, many political, but with nutrition there are some definite stand-outs. Our "food supply" is so far removed from the way it originated and I am hard pressed to consider most of it as "food." Unfortunately, if one does not know what they are truly consuming, one is exposed to potentially long-term health hazards. S.A.D is made up of processed foods with low nutrition value, chock full of sugar, bad fats, artificial dyes, and too many unhealthy carbs.

Damaged Fats, Sugar, and Toxins

These three culprits are the landmines one must avoid if at all possible. There are so many misconceptions, thanks largely in kind to our government, with regards to healthy and unhealthy fats. Most processed foods additionally contain sugar and toxins. Your body could be a well-oiled machine, but it is still unable to handle the constant onslaught of damaged fats, sugars, and toxins. Eventually this takes a great toll on one's short and long-term health if preventative measures are not acted upon.

There are specific nutritional suggestions which can immediately change your current state, completely transforming your future. The principles that work to accomplish this are not new, as it has only been in the past 100 years our dietary structure drastically changed for the sake of convenience. So many primitive cultures are free of America's chronic conditions and less than 100 years ago, the United States of America was considered one of them. Take into account what our great grandparents and beyond consumed and how they actually ate. Most of it was fresh, homemade, and unprocessed. All family members were present at the dinner table together, taking their time to eat and to socialize. Nothing compared to the frenetic rushing schedules of today, with time only to hover over tiny screens at a counter or sofa, mindlessly shoveling processed foods into our mouths, not cognizant many times of what we are even eating. This sadly is how we generally see nutrition approached as a family unit today.

My passion and focus have primarily been on the practical tools, resources, and tips to walk along side clients, guiding them through the various changes. The foods we consume to maintain a healthy diet and body have been historically successful, but nowadays, we do not even recognize what has become "normal" food in most double income families.

To avoid the three dangers of damaged fats, sugars, and toxins, there are easy basic changes to consider, regardless of age, gender, genetic background, or medical history.

Simple and Basic Healthy Changes

Fat – Consider consuming more healthy fats and eliminate damaged fats. Healthy fats include coconut oil, avocado oil, olive oil, flax oil (do not heat) butter, nuts/seeds, and fats from naturally raised animals. Examples of damaged fats would be vegetable oil, corn oil, canola oil, safflower oil, margarine, soybean oil, and cottonseed oil.

Protein – Focus on the quality of your proteins. When it comes to animal products, do your best to select organic, naturally raised foods vs. commercially raised. Select 100% grass-finished (fed) beef, wild-caught fish, and pasture-raised chicken and eggs. I recommend avoiding pork and shellfish. Always avoid processed meat which contains nitrates or nitrites. Unless otherwise specified, this includes lunch meat, bacon, packaged meats, hot dogs, salami, and packaged or frozen meats.

Carbohydrates – Introduce more vegetables and eliminate refined grains, sugars, and moderate grains. Concerning information is continually being released in the past few years revealing how toxic gluten can be for our brains and bodies. It is present in just about everything processed unless otherwise stated. It is a protein found in rye, wheat, and barley, and used, as thickening and curdling agents under many different names.

The carbohydrates you need can be acquired from foods other than grains and, really, there are no known deficiencies attributed to a lack of grains in one's diet. Following the USDA's recommendations for the RDA (Recommended Daily Allowance) would fill up more than 1/4 of our plate each meal and is completely unnecessary. If you wish to consume grains, stick with whole/sprouted grains, and/or ancient grains such as quinoa, amaranth, millet, kamut, and spelt. For many, this category can be the most challenging, however, there are so many alternatives to traditional grains and natural sugars that you can be successful without feeling deprived.

Grain Alternatives

- **Cauliflower** – Can be mashed to replace mashed potatoes, or "riced" for a rice replacement, or blended to thicken soups or sauces.
- **Spiralized Vegetables** – You can buy inexpensive kitchen gadgets that turn things like zucchini or squash into "noodles."

- **Almond Flour** – My favorite substitute for baking and replacing flour. It is a 1:1 conversion ratio and you will see tons of recipes for healthy bread and desserts on maxliving.com/healthy-recipes.
- **Garbanzo Bean Flour/Coconut Flour** – These are great blended in with almond flour or on their own. They are a little harder to work with because they are not an exact 1:1 conversion ratio, but certainly another great alternative for you to have available.
- **Cassava Flour** – There are oodles of commercial products out on the market which contain cassava flour to replace things like crackers and tortillas/tortilla chips.

Sugar Alternatives

Avoid – White sugar, turbinado sugar, agave syrup, corn syrup, all artificial sweeteners, and cane syrup.

Natural sweeteners – Use in moderation, eliminating all together if blood sugar is a concern; try dried fruits like dates, banana puree, and whole apple sauce.

Sugar alcohols – like xylitol (which FYI is very toxic to dogs and cats), erythritol, and maltitol, I advise to use in moderation. They may also cause digestive discomfort in some people.

Lakanto/Monk Fruit Sweetener – use as a 1:1 replacement for sugar.

Although these changes can be a challenge for many being so entrenched in the Standard American Diet, it can be done! It takes commitment and a willingness to change and I can encourage you from experience, even baby steps in these positive directions can have dramatic results.

Toxins

We are becoming more aware how significantly the role of genetics impacts our health. Just as fingerprints clearly identify one person out of hundreds of millions, so does our unique DNA structure. Because of these variations, we age differently, suffer from allergies others might not, have many different blood types, and contain pre-dispositions to genetic disorders and diseases others do not. If we continually expose ourselves to toxic dangers both nutritionally and environmentally, it can further erode our genetic pre-dispositions, allowing genetic related diseases such as MS or Parkinson's to rear their ugly heads later in life.

There is a highly unknown but fairly common genetic SNP (Single Nucleotide Polymorphism) called MTHFR–Methylenetetrahydrofolate Reductase–that is quickly gaining attention in understanding what can impact our genetics, affecting us long term. Most are completely unaware they have this genetic variation as doctors are just starting to understand, research, and learn about this sensitive, silent genetic destroyer. It is an enzyme which stimulates folic acid by turning it to folate. Folic acid in supplements are considered toxic if one has this SNP, so a bio-advanced "Folinic Acid" is recommended with B-12 once you have had verification from your doctor through testing that you possess these SNP's. They indicate significant pre-dispositioned sensitivity to toxins in foods, vaccines, alcohol, sugar, artificial dyes, amalgams, chemicals, water, body lotions, etc, which can mysteriously affect one's physical and mental health if not diagnosed properly. Individuals with this SNP should definitely avoid gluten.

Basic Meal Suggestions

Be sure to visit maxliving.com/healthy-recipes for hundreds of healthy, easy ideas and delicious recipes.

Breakfast Suggestions

- **Eggs** – Invest in free-range, organic eggs; try to find locally raised.
- **Mini Omelet Muffins** – Mix free-range, organic eggs, tomatoes, onions, spinach, etc. and bake in greased muffin tins.
- **Grapefruit**
- **Salad** – Be creative! A fruit salad is a great idea for breakfast!

- **Avocado** - Add to eggs, salad, wild-caught smoked salmon, smoothies, or enjoy alone.
- **Turkey Bacon** (nitrite-free, sugar-free)
- **Grain-Free Granola** (recipe on maxliving.com/healthy-recipes)

Lunch Suggestions

- **Salad** – Mix and match your favorite healthy ingredients. Purchase a bottle of extra-virgin olive oil and bottle of apple-cider vinegar to mix as a dressing. Top with a protein. Try free-range, organic eggs, free-range, organic chicken, or grass-fed steak, and top it off by adding some healthy fats like avocados, walnuts, etc.
- Quality protein source and abundant amounts of organic veggies.

Dinner Suggestions

- **Salad** – topped with source of protein. Again, try to add a healthy fat.
- Quality protein source. Abundant amounts of organic veggies.

Soups – Check ingredients on cans—ensure gluten-free—or make a couple of batches for the freezer, especially to have prepared when the baby arrives.

Snacks

- **Coconut Flakes**
- **Raw Almonds** – Other nuts and seeds are also a good option.
- **Celery Sticks** – With oil and vinegar or with almond butter.
- **Avocado** – Whole or smashed—with organic salsa or wild-caught smoked salmon.
- **Granny Smith Apples** – Alone or with almond butter, and in moderation.
- **Raw Veggies** – With or without dip.
- **Kale Chips** – In your oven or dehydrator. Store bought versions are available but expensive.
- **Grass-Fed Beef Jerky** – Homemade is easy! Just slice grass-fed beef very thin and marinate in gluten-free tamari or liquid aminos, garlic powder, red pepper flakes, or any other spices you prefer and dehydrate.

- **Chocolate Bark** – Must keep cool.
- **Trail Mix** – Combine raw nuts/seeds, coconut flakes, etc.
- **Organic Olives**
- **Hummus with Veggies** – Check ingredients if purchased.
- **Hard Boiled Eggs**
- **Grain-Free Crackers or Cereals**
- **Apple Flax Muffins** – recipe on maxliving.com/healthy-recipes

Drinks

- **Water** – Flavor with flavored stevia, lemon, lime, etc. for a bit of variety
- **Coconut Water**

Tips for Eating Out

- **Make friends with your server** – Briefly share what you hope to accomplish, as many times your server will come up with some creative ideas, discussing them one on one with the chef in order to accommodate you.
- **Scan the menu** – Look for substitutions or items you can pull together for a meal. Typically, you can look at menus online to provide more time and help make wise decisions before you go out.
- **Skip the sauce** – Sometimes there are entrees and sides you can order without the sauces, sugars, gluten, etc. Ask for a grilled chicken breast without sauce, and two sides of vegetables instead.
- **Ask for extra lemons** – Squeeze over your food if eliminating sauces, as they are a great way to add a punch of flavor.
- **Ask for olive oil or butter** – Often restaurants will have these items but cook them in vegetable oil, shortening, etc. Simply ask them to cook your food in olive oil or butter.
- **Salads** – build your own. Look through the menu and create your own concoction.
- **Make your own lemonade** – Ask for water and lemons, adding a little stevia.
- **Use olive oil and vinegar** – Instead of calorie-laden dressings, mix these two, or combining olive oil and lemons is another good fresh option.

- **Ask for avocado** – Many restaurants have them and they are a great way to consume good fats while you are out, and will fill you up as well.
- **Take your healthy condiments with you** – Keep a good quality Himalayan salt, and a small leak proof container of olive oil/vinegar for dressing in your purse or small travel bag to have on hand when you eat out.

Simple, Go-To Recipes

Preparing vegetables or a combination of vegetables is as simple as sautéing, grilling, baking, or steaming and seasoning to taste. These recipes and others are also available at the back of the book or at maxliving.com/healthy-recipes. All serving sizes can be adjusted online as well!

- Hummus
- Zesty Lemon Quinoa
- Blasted Cauliflower
- Green Beans with Walnuts
- Max Energy Bars

- Braised Fennel
- Brussels Sprouts Sautée
- Tahini Kale
- Stuffed Mushrooms
- Chili Zucchini Mash

Main Dishes

- Tortilla Chip Casserole
- Salmon Almondine
- Meatloaf
- Chicken Asparagus Marsala
- Mini Quiches
- Asian Turkey Lettuce Wraps
- Chili
- Chicken Salad
- Cod Provencal
- One Pan Balsamic Chicken and Vegetables
- Grass-fed Steaks
- Turkey Stuffed Acorn Squash
- Tex Mex Casserole
- Swedish Meatballs
- Chicken Soup

- Tex Mex Soup
- Loaded Cauliflower Bake
- Homemade Broth
- Chicken Spideini
- Cabbage Steaks
- Shepherd's Pie
- Pasta Salad
- Chicken Wings
- Spaghetti Squash with Beef Ragu
- Lasagna
- Vegetable Minestrone Soup
- Smoked Salmon Hash
- Philly Cheesecake Stuffed Peppers
- White Turkey Chili

Desserts/Baked Items

- No Bake Cheesecake
- Grainless Strawberry Bread
- Berry Parfaits
- Strawberry Fat Bombs
- Banana Bread

Beverages

- Max Fitterade
- Green Smoothie
- Pistachio Smoothie
- Berry Smoothie
- Mason Jar Cobblers
- Chocolate Chip Cookies
- Strawberry Gelato
- Protein Packed Brownies
- Chia Seed Pudding
- Cinnabites

Nutraceuticals During Pregnancy

Proper nutrition is vital during pregnancy, and you will observe specific nutritional recommendations throughout this book. While we never look at nutraceuticals as a replacement for a poor diet, there are specific nutraceuticals that are extremely beneficial during your pregnancy and beyond.

Before stopping or adding any supplements to your daily regiment, always discuss first with your Holistic Primary Care Physician and MaxLiving Doctor (See appendix).

MaxLiving Prenatal Daily Essentials Packets contain a prenatal multivitamin, essential fatty acids, and a bone supporting nutraceutical to provide you with optimal nutrients before, during, and after pregnancy.

As mentioned earlier, nutritional testing is a very accurate way to understand exactly where you are deficient. This helps determine what supplements you should be taking, and in what quantities. Your MaxLiving doctor can provide more information about specific testing for your needs.

Never take poor quality, sub-standard supplements, whether pregnant or not, as they can contain gluten, toxins, and be potentially dangerous.

Also, never go through any type of detoxification or take any detox products while you are pregnant or nursing.

For more information on MaxLiving products, visit www.maxliving.com.

****

CHAPTER 3

Taking Care of Your Body During Pregnancy

Exercise During Pregnancy

Prior to embarking on any type of exercise program, always first consult with your Holistic Primary Care Physician to ensure even small amounts of exercise are acceptable.

Ideally, exercise has been an ongoing practice for you prior to pregnancy. Every woman should be exercising before, during, and after pregnancy as movement is essential to good health. It is very beneficial to exercise during your pregnancy as the birth process itself is extremely physical. The better shape you are in, the better prepared and easier time you will have moving through the birthing process. Exercising also enables you to bounce back at a quicker rate afterwards. A good rule of thumb is to modify what you are currently doing (i.e., do not start an exercise program new to you). If you are not currently exercising, it is advisable after consulting with your doctor to engage in low intensity/low impact movements such as walking and swimming.

The MaxT3 program (see appendix) is a wonderful way to stay active during your pregnancy. MaxT3 can be modified during your pregnancy, so consult with your MaxLiving Doctor.

Chiropractic Care During Pregnancy

Pregnancy is physically demanding and it is vital your spine and nervous system be functioning at 100% capacity. The Chiropractic doctor will look for subluxations, which are mechanical disturbances to the normal alignment of the spine leading to disruption of the nervous system. These misalignments can interfere with signals flowing from the brain, down the spinal column to every nerve and organ of the body, affecting proper alignment of the pelvis, and joint dysfunction. Many pregnant women find significant relief from symptoms such as heartburn, nausea, constipation, pubic pain, sleep, etc. after receiving chiropractic care.

It is estimated 50% of pregnant women will experience back pain at some point during pregnancy. Chiropractic treatment can alleviate pain by taking pressure off the nerves and can help pregnant women avoid the use of painkillers, which can trigger unwanted side effects for mother and baby. A report in the Journal of the American Chiropractic Association showed 75% of pregnant women who received chiropractic treatment experienced pain relief.[7]

During the third trimester, the hormone Relaxin can increase, resulting in joints becoming loose, preparing for birth, which can decrease joint stability potentially altering posture. This can also contribute to back pain. Dr. Irvin Henderson, MD (a member of the American Medical Association Board of Trustees) conducted a study that demonstrated how "women who received chiropractic adjustments in their third trimester were able to carry and deliver their child with much more comfort."[8]

Chiropractic care throughout pregnancy has also been shown to reduce labor time. In one study, Dr. Joan Fallon found first-time mothers averaged 25% shorter labor duration, while those on their second pregnancy or beyond had a 31% reduction in average labor time.[9] Our personal experience in a clinical setting has been women under chiropractic care report shorter labor times, less complications, and less medical interventions.

Tips to care for your spine and nervous system during pregnancy:

Regular visits to your MaxLiving doctor for adjustments.

As opposed to sitting straight up after resting or sleeping, rise by turning on to your side, bending and bringing your knees up, pushing yourself up with your arm instead.

Wear comfortable shoes and avoid wearing heels.

For infrequent lifting, keep it under 20-30 lbs. For an hour or more of lifting, keep under 15 lbs.

Instead of turning or swiveling at the hips, move your body in one plane. For example, to get out of a car, open the door and turn your whole body towards the door, swinging your legs and upper body at the same time. Once your feet are on the ground, stand up.

Be very careful lifting or carrying older children. If this must take place, be sure to lift with your legs. Squat and lift rather than bending over. This can cause your back to round adding pressure to the lower back. Also, avoid habitually carrying children on one side/hip only.

Practice Kegel exercises to work on your pelvic floor muscles. Kegel exercises are also known as pelvic floor exercises. They help strengthen the muscles beneficial for pregnancy as well as bladder and bowel function. Many women experience bladder leakage, so Kegels are a great preventative and management technique.

Regular moderate exercise (after first consulting with your Holistic Primary Care Physician to ensure you are cleared for this activity).

Stretch often and frequently.

Hire a massage therapist regularly.

****

CHAPTER 4
First Trimester
Approximately 0-13 weeks

This is a very exciting time, especially if this is your first pregnancy! You will begin to notice your body changing and responding to the miracle of life. This is the opportune time to read through this entire book, have a notebook ready to write questions, and start journaling about your pregnancy, discussing goals and expectations with your spouse. As I mentioned in the beginning, your baby's brain and spinal cord are first to develop during this trimester, most other vital organs and systems will develop as well.

Staying on schedule with your chiropractic adjustments during the first trimester is critical to ensure a healthy pregnancy and delivery. Pregnant women many times use the SOS, "Sleep on Side", position. Therefore, sleep aids (wedges and rolls) are not recommended during pregnancy. You can always go back to this sleeping style after the delivery.

A MaxLiving Wobble Cushion may be used to loosen joints, nourish the discs, maintaining motion in the lumbar spine. A hanging traction unit can be used to do the same for the cervical spine.

If you already are experienced with MaxLiving's home exercise equipment, the continuation of these exercises should be determined by your MaxLiving Doctor.

What You May Be Feeling

You may be experiencing some nausea, but not necessarily. A good tip for averting nausea is to try to always keep something in your stomach. Eat small, frequent, healthy meals and snacks, readily available and with you at all times. Nuts and seeds are great protein snacks to keep on hand, and protein helps stave off hunger.

Hormonal changes will be occurring, so fatigue is something you may experience frequently. Expect to be more tired than usual as there is a significant increase in energy demand for your growing baby.

Losing a little weight is common. Do not be concerned about this unless weight loss is considerable and persists past the first trimester.

You may notice more frequent urination.

There may be some hip pain or discomfort and not uncommon as your body is preparing to deliver a baby. You may also notice ligaments stretching feeling like sharp pains in your uterus. A belly band can be a great addition to your wardrobe and help keep you in your regular clothes a little longer.

Mood swings might become more frequent as your hormones are increasing and you may feel more emotional or "out of control" than normal. If this is frequent, evaluate your diet as sugar, gluten, artificial dyes, or caffeine can further exacerbate your moods.

What You Should and Should Not Be Eating

Consider following the Core or Advanced Plan from the *"Align Your Health"* book (see appendix).

Ensure you have adequate protein intake as pregnancy considerably increases your need. Typically, one requires approximately 80g of protein daily by the second trimester. Almond butter is a healthy, quick and easy protein punch. Eat a couple of tablespoons right out of the jar first thing in the morning, or add it to a smoothie to start the day.

Drink plenty of water. Eight to twelve 8-oz. glasses of purified water a day would be a great start. Dehydration is the primary cause of pre-term labor, so don't overlook your need for water. Fill the same pitcher each day with your daily hydration requirements to help keep track of your daily hydration progress.

Always avoid processed meat, which contains nitrates or nitrites. This includes lunch meat with nitrates, bacon, packaged meat, hot dogs, salami, or packaged or frozen meats. Avoid pork and shellfish altogether.

Always avoid honey and all processed sugars. Any high natural sugar intake should be minimized too.

What to Expect if Choosing an OB-GYN Office and Hospital Birth

Always have an advocate with you and in the room at all times. It could be your spouse, bu it is advisable to also have a Doula to help you through the entire process, and their role will be explained shortly. Prepare to be faced with many decisions at doctor appointments. Carefully consider each of them, especially regarding ultrasounds and other testing. Once in labor and at the hospital, you are very vulnerable to hasty decisions and pressure by medical staff, because you are there on their time clock.

Ultrasound

One recommendation certain to be presented early on by medical staff is to have an ultrasound. Ultrasounds, sonograms, and Doppler use high-frequency sound waves to produce an image of the baby on a viewing screen or amplify the baby's heartbeat. They wish to determine how far along in pregnancy you are, and to use Doppler to hear the baby's heartbeat. You should note no studies have been conducted proving the safety of these devices, and the American Medical Association recommends against unnecessary exposure to high frequency waves from these devices.

Unnecessary ultrasound exposure includes the use of these devices to:

- Determine the sex of the baby.
- Determine gestational age (how many weeks old the baby is).
- Assess the size and growth of the baby.
- Confirm or rule out multiple pregnancies.
- Determine fetal presentation (position of baby in the womb).

Another study states, "Physicians should continue to be prudent about the use of ultrasound and perform the study only when medically necessary and when benefits outweigh the risk according to the American College of Radiology. The advice comes in the wake of recent findings by Yale researchers that link prenatal ultrasound exposure to brain damage."[10] Ultrasound energy is a high-frequency mechanical vibration which stimulates the fetus and can affect brain neurons. Use of ultrasound has also shown significantly higher intrauterine growth restriction and lower weight babies.[11] Since ultrasound is not a necessity, we recommend avoiding it or use sparingly at a bare minimum.

Many couples use ultrasound to determine the sex of the baby. While it is in our nature to want to plan ahead, to have a gender reveal party, and to decorate the baby's room, I am so thankful we waited to find out. Of course, it is every couple's choice, but I would suggest evaluating and researching this more prior to making a decision to find out. My husband always jokes, "if God wanted us to know, a mom's belly would turn pink or blue."

It was such a wonderful and memorable moment for Fred and I finding out at the actual delivery we had a son, then a daughter from the second pregnancy, and again a son from our third pregnancy.

The anticipation was all part of our birth experience. It is hard to describe the feeling but I cherish each of those three moments to this day.

3D and 4D Ultrasounds: These are very popular and make many parents happy because the images are much more detailed and are great keepsakes to share with your nanna and poppa to hang proudly on the fridge.

However, they are even more dangerous and there is no medical need for them. Even the FDA advises against them stating, "Ultrasounds can heat tissues and in some cases, produce very small bubbles or cavitation in some tissues."[12]

These types of ultrasounds put even more stress on the fetus than regular ultrasounds. Registered Sonographers know the technology and can better control the length and intensity of the session, as opposed to non-registered personnel. Again, please, do your research!

Lab Tests: Standard tests include anemia, blood type, sexually transmitted diseases, and a pap smear. These items listed are for "normal" pregnancies. If anything identified as "abnormal" is detected, more interventions/tests will typically be done.

What to Expect If You Have Chosen a Homebirth/Midwife/Doula

Midwives and Doulas monitor the physical, psychological, and social well-being of the mother throughout the childbearing cycle. Their duty is to provide the mother with individualized education, counseling, and prenatal care, offering continuous hands-on assistance during labor and delivery. They provide postpartum support, work to minimize technological medical interventions, identify women who require obstetrical attention, and make referrals to other appropriate medical personnel. Hiring either one or both will help ensure you have educated advocates truly in your corner with extensive experience, and most likely sharing and protecting your values. They generally help instill peace, comfort, and confidence.

Certified Midwife – Offers prenatal care (i.e., regular visits throughout your pregnancy) and are trained professionals who will be present at the birth and at checkups. The standard rate for a midwife in the year 2020 can range from $1500 - $5000 (See appendix).

Certified Doula – A labor coach very experienced with the stages of labor, wisely discerning how to coach women through natural deliveries. In the year 2020, the standard rate for a Doula can range in cost from $800 - $2500 (See appendix).

Looking Ahead

Vaccines

One major decision you will need to make is regarding vaccinations. While we are only discussing the First Trimester, please start to do your research now in order to arm yourself with knowledge and truth.

Once a vaccination has been administered, it cannot be undone. Please go to the Vaccine section of this book when you are ready to learn more on this crucial part of your birth plan.

Probiotic Gulp

It is very important to have flourishing healthy gut bacteria before you give birth. When your baby is born, their gut is completely sterile. The first colonization occurs as the baby passes through the birth canal and is why vaginal births are so important. This is critical for the establishment and strength of your baby's immune system moving forward.

Babies born via C-section miss this very important step, so it is advisable to take a swab of the mother's birth canal and put it in your baby's mouth right away. If the baby does not receive this first colonization, they are at an immediate disadvantage, vulnerable for a lifetime of negative health consequences such as asthma, allergies, and other autoimmune disorders.

Vaginal births can take much longer which is why doctors in recent years made history "pushing" (pun intended) – C-Sections – you are in their house and now fit better into their schedules.[13] C-Section births are taking place at an alarming rate compared to the past and babies are losing out on this precious bacterial commodity from their mother.

Another significant benefit of selecting vaginal birth is the "squeezing" that takes place while baby is passing through the birth canal. This seemingly inconsequential rite of passage – literally – helps force fluids out of the airway, eliminating the need for suctioning.

So, these are a few reasons why it is essential to attend to your own gut health by eliminating processed foods and the use of antibiotics as they can negatively affect your gut flora. Also, naturally fermented foods like barrel-cured organic sauerkraut, kimchi, unsweetened kefir, and kombucha are known to be wonderful in promoting healthy gut flora.

****

CHAPTER 5
Second Trimester
Approximately 14-27 weeks

During the second trimester, major events are transpiring within you concerning the development of your baby. This is the time development of the five senses takes place, including the ability to hear and distinguish voices,. During this time fingerprints, muscles, ligaments, facial features, hair, and eyes evolve. By the end of this Second Trimester, your baby's weight most likely will have doubled.

What You May Be Feeling:

Quickening – The moment you first feel your baby move, it will give the sensation of a "flutter."

Expect additional body expansion. Weight gain should be between 3 to 5 pounds per month and your belly should grow a few centimeters per week.

Typically, if nausea was common, it usually subsides at this time, but not always. Make sure you are eating enough protein every day and drinking plenty of water. Remember to always keep healthy snacks on hand and something in your stomach.

The "nesting" phenomena begins. Expect bursts of additional energy, preparing and setting things up for the arrival of your baby.

One significant morphological change your body will experience is the oxygen demand increase of the growing fetus. Your lung capacity increases, resulting in a "spreading" of the rib cage. It is not uncommon for women to experience thoracic (chest or back area) pain of varying natures. These mechanical changes can result in subluxation (misalignment) of the spine and rib head (where the rib attaches to the spine) issues that can be extremely painful. I actually experienced this painful issue with each of my pregnancies, and was very thankful Fred was a chiropractor as at times it felt like a knife sticking out of my back.

What You Should and Should Not Be Eating:

Consider following the Core or Advanced Plan from the *"Align Your Health"* book. In addition, these are a few more Second Trimester recommendations:

Increase your caloric intake approximately 300 calories/day.

Maintain your protein intake to 80 g daily.

Drink plenty of water! Drink at least eight 8-12 oz. glasses of purified water per day. It is important to remember – dehydration is the primary cause of pre-term labor!

What to Expect if You Have Chosen to Use an OB-GYN Office and Hospital Birth

You will be offered an Alpha-fetoprotein (AFP) test to screen for possible neural tube defects (such as Spinal Bifida) and Downs Syndrome. If you are over the age of 35, you will be offered amniocentesis to diagnose possible fetal abnormalities. This is not medically necessary and carries considerable risks, including miscarriage. There is also risk of infection, leaking of amniotic fluid, cramping, and actually injecting the baby with a needle.

I highly discourage these tests. If you are not planning on terminating your pregnancy, the AFP test then serves no purpose. Historically it has very high false positive rates as well, leading to unnecessary stress and anxiety for expectant parents and their extended families. There are many dangers to amniocentesis and they are very intrusive. Please talk to your MaxLiving Doctor before agreeing to subject yourself and your baby to either of these tests.

What to Expect if You Have Chosen a Homebirth/Midwife/Doula

As I explained in the First Trimester, midwives and doulas monitor the physical, psychological and social well-being of the mother throughout the childbearing cycle, providing the mother with individualized education, counseling, and prenatal care. They also offer continuous hands-on assistance during labor and delivery.

Your midwife may start palpating the baby by pressing lightly around your stomach, or may use a fetoscope (a non-invasive listening device similar to a stethoscope) to hear the baby's heartbeat.

Massage

This is a great time to start regular massages, but not before the second trimester. Make sure your massage therapist is certified in prenatal massage. Some may have a table with a hole in it to accommodate your growing belly, others may ask you lay on your side with a pillow. Massage benefits can include:

- Elimination of waste, which stimulates the lymphatic and circulatory systems.
- Blood pressure control, which aides in circulation.
- Reduction of muscle discomfort, tightness, cramping, stiffness, and sciatica.
- Hormonal balancing, which reduces stress hormone levels.
- Headache and sinus relief due to increased blood flow.
- Edema reduction, which stimulates lymphatic drainage.
- Optimal nourishment by improved blood circulation to you and the baby.
- Increased flexibility through relaxed muscles, tendons, and ligaments.
- Increased relaxation, which helps you sleep better.
- During labor, a massage can help reduce low back discomfort.
- After birth, a massage can help with recovery.[14]

****

CHAPTER 6

Third Trimester
Approximately 28–40 weeks

You certainly will know by now you have life growing inside with all the movement occurring from the baby. Your baby will also gain about 1/2 a pound per week, making the movement much more noticeable as he or she expands. At this point your baby's lungs are fully mature and brain neurons are developing rapidly.

Delivery time is quickly approaching, so enjoy every last minute of your final trimester.

What You May Be Feeling:
- Increased movement
- Increased fatigue
- Cramps/ligaments stretching
- Lack of comfort
- Frequent urination
- Swelling in the feet and ankles
- Pelvic separation that can be painful

What You Should and Should Not Be Eating
Consider following the Core or Advanced Plan from the *"Align Your Health"* book. In addition to the First and Second Trimester recommendations:

Towards the end of the Third Trimester you may slightly reduce your protein intake.

Keep hydration levels very high.

Avoid giant pasta dinners at the end of the third trimester (refer back to my birth story).

What to Expect if You Have Chosen to use an OB-GYN Office and Hospital Birth

Around 26 weeks, medical personnel will usually recommend a glucose-tolerance test to determine your susceptibility for gestational diabetes. This procedure entails consuming an excessively sugary drink and testing your blood sugar. This test is discouraged, as the "drink" used for the test contains highly toxic ingredients. The ingredients of the popular brand EasyDex by Aromed are: "water, dextrose natural flavoring, modified food starch, glycerol ester of wood rosin, brominated soybean oil, FD&C Yellow, Sodium Hexametaphosphate, BHA, and .10% Sodium benzoate."[15]

Dextrose is a processed sugar from corn and bominated oils have been shown to build up in the body and has numerous toxic effects.

A much better option is a glucometer to measure blood glucose levels. These tools are relatively inexpensive and significantly safer for you and your baby.

Guidelines for glucose levels:

If you opt to use a glucometer, guidelines for glucose levels are as follows:

> Fasting blood glucose (first thing in the morning) = 86 or lower
> 1 hour after eating = 140 or lower
> 2 hours after eating = 120 or lower
> 3 hours after eating = back to fasting level [16]

Around 37 weeks, the doctor will begin examining your cervix to determine your progress. Around 39 weeks, possibly earlier, expect the doctor to ask if you would like early induction. I highly discourage the inducing of labor, as so often the process for determining a due date is flawed and it is perfectly safe to go several weeks beyond your due date. Induction increases labor pains, often leading to other interventions, especially epidurals and C-sections.

What to Expect if You Have Chosen a Homebirth / Midwife / Doula

As in the First and Second Trimester, they will continue to monitor the physical, psychological and social well-being of the mother throughout the childbearing cycle. They will provide the mother with individualized education, counseling, and prenatal care. Your midwife will palpate to see how the baby is positioned in the uterus.

Start perineal massage around 34 weeks. Perineal massage is extremely helpful in reducing pain and preventing the need for an episiotomy. Referring back to the birth of our three children, I did not tear, nor was I pressured to have an episiotomy.

For more information on how to learn this massage technique, please refer to the appendix.

Women who opt for episiotomies often experience:

- Extension of the incision
- Increased pain and discomfort
- Difficult and prolonged healing
- Increased risk of infection
- Increased pain during intercourse (short and long-term)
- Increased bowel incontinence
- Decreased sexual function
- Pressure from medical staff to have C-sections for future deliveries

****

CHAPTER 7
Labor & Delivery

There are several things to consider well in advance of your labor and delivery. If you have chosen a hospital birth, it is advisable to stay at home until your labor has sufficiently progressed. Wait until your contractions are fairly close together before you go to the hospital. Other important considerations include epidurals, baby presentation, type of birth, episiotomy, extraction techniques, C-sections, and circumcision.

Birth Options

A top priority on your "To-Do" list is to decide how and what birthing method of delivery you wish to proceed with as soon as possible. There are many options available, so I encourage you to consider them all so you can make an educated decision on what you feel is best for your family.

Traditional OB-GYN/Hospital Birth

This is the common choice for most Americans. As was discussed earlier, I highly encourage a natural childbirth process with minimal medical interventions, so selecting a hospital setting can be a challenge. This is not to say it will not work, however, it is essential to have a concrete "birth plan" in place with your hospital.

Midwives tend to be a bit more open to natural childbirth, so it is a good idea to find an OB-GYN practice with midwives. It is also imperative to have a good relationship with the doctors and midwives at the office you choose. A hospital setting will dramatically increase the potential for medical interventions, labor inductions, and C-sections.

Many people are afraid something may occur during the childbirth process if they choose a home birth or a birthing center. They believe there "might" be a need for services available in a hospital setting. This is a valid concern, but read on to learn actual statistics and how this can be approached and handled. Costs can vary, but at a minimum in the year 2020, a hospital visit will start around $6,000 and goes up from there, so plan on spending at least $10,000 for the birth.

I cannot encourage you and your spouse enough to attend a natural childbirth class during your pregnancy. Also, I recommend selecting a Doula to be present at the birth to help you through the labor process.

Certified Midwife – They offer prenatal care (i.e., regular visits throughout your pregnancy) and are trained professionals who will be present at the birth and at checkups.

Certified Doula – A very experienced labor coach who knows how to coach women through the stages of labor and natural deliveries.

Birthing Center – Depending where you live, you may have access to birthing centers which are typically more holistically based. Most birthing centers will not augment (induce) labor, use monitoring, or perform epidural procedures. Many birthing centers are affiliated with hospitals, which can increase chances of medical interventions, so be sure to research thoroughly (See appendix).

Home Birth Information

Having a home birth is a very personal decision. Home births significantly reduce chances of unnecessary interventions and can be fantastic, personal, and intimate experiences for you and your family, as you control the environment. Many women who select home births describe the events as extremely spiritual, allowing them to be completely in tune with their babies and the miracle of the birthing process. Many home births include water birth, which also presents various options as well. Although this may seem frightening to some, I suggest seeking out women who have experienced home births. Research shows home births are extremely safe, providing parents much more control over their decisions.[17] Home birthing is an acceptable alternative to hospital confinement for pregnant women, leading to reduced medical interventions. I encourage you to research this option thoroughly and remember, pregnancy is not an illness to be "treated", but rather experienced with you and your wishes at the helm.

The American Public Health Association wrote about "recognizing the evidence that births to healthy mothers, who are not considered at medical risk after comprehensive screening by trained professionals, can occur safely in various settings, including out-of-hospital birth centers and homes. Therefore, APHA Supports efforts to increase access to out-of-hospital maternity care services...". Plus according to the American Journal of Public Health there is "Increasing Access to Out-of-Hospital Maternity Care Services through State-Regulated and Nationally-Certified Direct-Entry Midwives (Policy Statement)". American Journal of Public Health, Vol 92, No. 3, March 2002. [18]

Additionally, a study from Oxford University Press stated, "several methodologically sound observational studies have compared the outcomes of planned home-births (irrespective of the eventual place of birth) with planned hospital births for women with similar characteristics. A meta-analysis of these studies showed no maternal mortality, and no statistically significant differences in perinatal mortality risk in either direction."[19]

In addition "the largest study of planned, Midwife-led home birth in the U.S. to date, reported outcomes for nearly 17,000 women who went in to labor intending to deliver at home between 2004 and 2009." [20]

Safe Outcomes with Positive Benefits

- High rate of completed home birth (89.1%)
- High rate of vaginal birth (93.6%)
- High rate of completed vaginal birth after cesarean (VBAC; 87.0%)
- Low intrapartum and neonatal fetal death rate overall: 2.06 per 1000 intended home births (includes all births) 1.61 per 1000 intended home births excluding breech, VBAC, twins, gestational diabetes, and preeclampsia.
- Low rate of low APGAR scores
- Extremely high rate of breastfeeding (97.7%) at 6 weeks" [21]

I also like to point out women have been giving birth throughout the centuries outside of a hospital setting. While some may argue mothers and babies suffered because of a lack of medical interventions, the case can also be made that many mothers and babies now suffer due to unnecessary medical interventions. For a normal pregnancy, which most are, a home birth is a perfectly natural and acceptable choice.

Brace yourself prior to researching United States infant mortality rates, as they are absolutely staggering. With the majority of women selecting hospital births and easy access to advanced medical treatments, this number does not match up to the theory "more is better" in terms of medical intervention compared to home births.

Water Birth

There are many benefits to choosing a water birth. This option allows the baby to move from the birth canal into an environment very similar to being in the womb and is far less of a shock for the baby. The warmth of the water provides pain relief for the mother, allowing her to be in a sitting position, capitalizing on gravity buoyancy. Water births have also revealed a reduction or elimination of tearing during birthing. There are many options for water births at home, including right in a bathtub, or in an inflatable birthing pool.

Hypno-Birth

Another option is to seek out a Hypno-Birthing instructor in your area. The premise of a Hypno-Birth is to embrace that a woman's body designed to give birth, and to completely trust in that process. You will learn how to tap into your natural birthing instincts effectively, achieving a level of relaxation and elimination of fear. There are several great online resources available for you to explore.

The Truth About Due Dates

One of the very first things established at the doctor's office is a "due date." It is human nature to want a timeline, and general guidelines are just fine. However, many expectant mothers, their families, doctors, nurses, and midwives put far too much emphasis on this "due date." It has been ingrained in our psyche that a normal pregnancy is 40 weeks using "Naegele's Rule." This was based on a biblical reference that pregnancy lasts approximately 10 lunar months, taking into account the time between when Mary was visited by the Angel Gabriel and the day of Jesus' birth. The calculation uses 28 days for one lunar month, making pregnancy a gestational period of 280 days. An exact lunar month is 29.53 days, which would add about 15 days to the readily accepted 280 days. It is estimated if a woman receives no medical interventions, 50 to 80% of the time, her pregnancy will go beyond 40 weeks and result in a perfectly normal delivery.

Many practitioners will use ultrasound, attempting to keep tabs on the due date, but there is mounting research when ultrasound is used, it becomes more inaccurate as the weeks go on. So, this procedure is really not all that reliable of a means either, not to mention safety of ultrasounds we discussed earlier in the book. It is important to note even the American College of Obstetricians and Gynecologists does not recommend intervening during a normal pregnancy before 41 weeks.[22] Therefore, when recommendations are made contradicting this, you can be armed with accurate information.

A much better method determining your estimated due date requires diligence tracking your menstrual cycle. If you are actively trying to get pregnant, keep a journal of your cycle. If you know the first date of your last menstrual period, the formula is simple and based on a reputable study conducted in 1990. It demonstrated first-time mother's pregnancies lasted an average of 288 days (41 weeks + 1 day). Women who previously gave birth had an average gestation of 283 days (40 weeks + 3 days).

Here is the calculation:

First-time mothers: Last menstrual period date minus 3 months + 15 days
Second pregnancy and beyond: Last menstrual period date minus 3 months + 10 days.[23]

Always keep in mind your body was created to naturally know what it is doing and there is no magic number. As long as everything is going along as expected, a birth can go well past a due date without complications. Do not be pressured into inducing labor based on a faulty calculation or scare tactics. Especially if there is no deterioration of baby's environment or other signs and symptoms of distress, be patient, trusting your body to do exactly what it was created to do.

Epidurals

Between 50 and 70% of American women are subjected to an epidural during delivery. Epidurals are labeled as safe, quick, and effective for laboring mothers. Unfortunately, these soon-to-be mom and dads are just not appropriately informed of what an epidural is and what the possible side effects may be. Epidurals are usually a combination of two opiates, Fentanyl and Bupivacaine. Fentanyl has 80 times the potency of morphine. Bupivacaine has been linked to tremors, blurred vision, central nervous system depression, seizures, loss of conscience, and respiratory depression. [24] The two medications together form an extremely potent combination which decreases and may wholly inhibit releasing life-giving oxytocin. [25]

During the natural process of labor, oxytocin – a naturally occurring hormone – is released in response to the stretching of the uterus and cervix. Oxytocin is also released from nipple stimulation during breastfeeding, and helps with the birth process, bonding, and milk production. A woman's hormones are intended to help orchestrate the bodily process of pushing out and positioning the baby. However, once an epidural is introduced, a woman's system (including the uterus, cervix, and pelvic muscle sling) becomes too relaxed to complete this work on its own. The medications muffle normal contractions and can often slow down or stop contractions altogether, as natural signals within a woman's body are no longer loud and clear. When labor slows, it leaves the mother highly susceptible to other additional medical interventions. It is very common for a labor progressing along nicely to slow down or cease once an epidural is given. This can ironically lead to the introduction of Pictocin – a synthetic version of Oxytocin – yes, the naturally occurring hormone, just diminished by the epidural. Induction can throw off the delicate, natural balance of the labor and delivery process. Labor can become rapid, which results in more violent and aggressive contractions, often leading to a C-section.

Keeping all of your faculties together during labor and delivery will help you with breathing, keeping you mentally focused, and supporting your intuition concerning pushing the baby through the birth canal. Yes, there is pain, but it is the pain which helps the process move forward. If you do decide to get an epidural, please fully understand possible ramifications by taking necessary precautions. When you have accurate and critical facts concerning medical procedures, make conscientious and informed choices for the care of you and your baby. The use of a supportive spouse, midwives, and doulas has also been shown to improve the probability of an un-medicated, natural birth.

The World Health Organization says: "Epidural Analgesia is one of the most striking examples of the medicalization of normal birth, transforming a physiological event into a medical procedure." [26]

Here are some of the risks and complications that can occur and are associated with the use of epidural analgesia:

- Hormonal Interference with oxytocin release – potentially forcing the need for Pitocin augmentation.
- Drop in blood pressure – causing lack of proper oxygenation to your body and possible shock.
- Stopped or slowed progression of natural labor – potentially leading to increased medical interventions and complications.
- Urinary tract/bladder infections and dysfunctions – caused by catheter use during epidural.
- Beta-endorphins which help the laboring mother receive natural pain relief, are inhibited, these hormones were created to help your body naturally deal with stress and pain.
- Maternal fever – medical providers will typically separate mother from baby in order to check for infection. This can include a septic workup, which could also mean antibiotics will be prescribed.
- Spinal headache – requiring extra days of rest or a possible blood patch to block the insertion hole of the needle.
- Risk of hemorrhage – twice as likely to happen with an epidural.
- Breastfeeding setbacks – very common for mothers who have epidurals. Drugs administered during labor can tremendously affect a newborn's feeding behavior. Not only can the onset of breastfeeding be delayed, studies show mothers who have epidurals have a shorter duration of breastfeeding. Mothers who have epidurals and Pitocin can have significant prolactin (milk production) delays.
- Heart problems – Mothers can experience bradycardia (slow heart rate) and can cause suppression of electrical heart activity, serious dissociation of the heart chambers, causing the heart to stop.

- Epidural use – often leads to baby's delivery requiring use of forceps and vacuum delivery of the baby.
- Increased episiotomy incidences – due to mother's inability to push the baby out effectively.
- Long-term back pain at the injection site.
- Substantial muscle damage of the pelvic floor sling (levator trauma) – caused by the inability to push effectively.
- Sphincter injury – several studies have concluded a high increase and likelihood of this type of injury to your bottom because of the failure to push effectively.
- Thrombosis of an artery from the epidural injection.
- Cranial nerve – paralysis.
- Hematoma caused by blood gathering in the spinal cord area.

Once again, I highly recommend researching, practicing your due diligence, understanding comprehensively the risks and benefits. Make a solid logical decision based on facts and common sense.

"I don't have any science or medical research to support this notion, but I believe women were giving birth even before epidurals were invented." Dr. Fred Roberto.

Breech Presentation

A breech presentation of a baby is usually the result of uterine constraint. There are several different types of breech presentations, and all can result in successful deliveries. However, it is ideal to have the baby in the head-first position. If your baby presents breech before birth, I recommend finding a Chiropractor who can perform the "Webster Technique" to help promote the baby to turn in a more desirable presentation. The success rate of this procedure is just over 80% [27] and my husband, Dr. Fred Roberto, has had great success with this technique over his 20 years in practice. One patient came in to his office, bruises all over her abdomen from a nurse practitioner who had manually tried to "turn" her breeched baby. My husband used the Webster Technique and told her to come back the next day for another treatment. She never showed up for her appointment, but later returned his call to update she had given birth that night after the Webster adjustment. She shared she had given birth to a head – first baby in the shower at her home. It happened so quickly she was unable to make it to the hospital.

Performance of the Webster Technique involves analysis of the relationship of the bones of the pelvis and a two-step correction of misaligned neuro-biomechanics through 1. the use of a light force chiropractic adjustment of the sacrum and pelvis, and 2. involving analysis and relief of specific abdominal muscle tension or spasm. Both steps are intended to relieve the musculoskeletal causes of intrauterine constraint that may lead to a C-section delivery.

Vaginal Birth

The body's natural birthing process is vaginal delivery, in which a woman's body was specifically created to perform the grand entrance of a baby's birth. As long as there is no medical interference, just at the right time, a woman's body does exactly what it is supposed to during labor and delivery. Your baby will come out to greet you and the world once they have completed their developing and growing. When labor begins, a hormone we just discussed called oxytocin increases. Among many things, this hormone stimulates contractions, which helps to open and dilate the cervix, contracting the uterus and moving the baby down through the birth canal. It also helps to expel the placenta, limit bleeding, and stimulate milk let down for nursing. As mentioned earlier, when Pitocin (the artificial representation of oxytocin) is given during the labor process, the medication hinders these processes from taking place naturally, possibly prolonging the birth process.

As I explained in the First Trimester's chapter, it is very important to have flourishing gut bacteria before you give birth. When your baby is born, their gut is completely sterile and immunity needs to be built. This first colonization occurs as the baby passes through the birth canal, and is critical for the strength of your baby's immune system.
Babies born via C-section miss this very important step. If the baby does not receive this first colonization, it can set them up for a lifetime of illness.

Episiotomy

Many have been led to believe episiotomies are necessary and part of a normal in birth, but you should know the risks. It is advisable to avoid having one, even if you end up with a natural tear. Think about a piece of cotton fabric and imagine trying to tear it without cutting it first. When a piece of fabric is torn, the tear is somewhat jagged, and takes considerably more effort to pull apart to create a large tear. Now imagine cutting a little slit in the fabric with a pair of scissors, and tearing it with the help of the already cut slit. You will find the tear is much cleaner (not jagged) and takes much less force to split apart. The skin of your perineum is similar. A natural tear will be able to heal more quickly and more fully as opposed to a tear where an incision is made.[28]

Vacuum Extraction/Forceps

These are often used when emergency situations arise (either mother or baby is in distress), and are usually a by-product of previous other medical interventions. The best way to avoid these is to be proactive, eliminating the possibility of an emergency situation to occur. I highly discourage the use of vacuum extraction or forceps for several reasons. According to a 2009 study in the Annual Review of Biomedical Engineering, approximately 12 pounds of pressure is applied to the head of the baby during a normal contraction, and 27 pounds of pressure is applied when a woman pushes during a contraction. When a vacuum device is applied, there is an additional force of 25 pounds or even more. This means there can be upwards of 52 pounds of pressure with each push. [29]

If a vacuum extraction procedure was used on your baby, contact a chiropractor for evaluation as soon as possible (see appendix). The chances of a doctor using the vacuum extraction are increased when an epidural thwarts the labor process. Be sure to include your stance on this topic in your birth plan.

When a human is delivering a baby with his/her hands, there are sensory receptors in the fingers which receive stimuli from the baby. Mechanoreceptors sense pressure, force, vibrations, and textures.

Proprioceptors detect position, movement, and spatial awareness (where things are in space and time and in relation to one another). Vacuum extraction devices and forceps, of course, do not have the ability to feel this. The use of mechanical devices increase the risk of injury to the baby. Babies are meant to be pushed out of the birth canal, not pulled.

Are you starting to see how one decision in the beginning starts to impact another, and then another, and how quickly a domino effect can take place?

C-section

Cesarean sections in the U.S. are at an all-time high. According to the CDC, cesarean births account for 32% of total births as of 2018. However, approximately 20% of hospitals have cesarean rates over 30%. [30] In a 2013 study, "working with 2009 data from 593 US hospitals nationwide, we found that cesarean rates varied tenfold across hospitals, from 7.1 percent to 69.9 percent. Even for women with lower-risk pregnancies, in which more limited variation might be expected, cesarean rates varied fifteen-fold, from 2.4 percent to 36.5 percent." [31]

The World Health Organization (WHO) states any time a country's cesarean section rate rises above 15%, the dangers of a C-section surgery outweigh its "lifesaving" benefits. While there is sometimes a need for this medical intervention, it has become far more "routine" than necessary. Many times, doctors and health professionals recommend C-section's far too quickly. In fact, shockingly enough, many families actually request C-sections to know exactly when their baby will be born. Or, have the misconception it is an easier process than experiencing the natural birth path through a vaginal birth.

C-section's are considered major surgery and should not be approached lightly. Unfortunately, medical personnel many times can unintentionally instill fear in parents if one is not well armed with truth. This emotional pull can wrongly influence the laboring parents, who agree too quickly to a C-section. Research shows babies born by C-section are at higher risk for health complications than with vaginal births. [32]

Also, cranial molding or "resetting" of the skull is absent during a C-section, and remember, exposure to beneficial bacteria (the probiotic gulp) is not available naturally when babies are not born vaginally. If you have a C-section, swab the birth canal and put it into the baby's mouth immediately to ensure proper gut colonization (refer to First Trimester/ Looking Ahead section). Both cranial molding and gut colonization are major benefits of vaginal births.

"Since 1990, C-sections have more than tripled from about 6 percent of all births to 21 percent, three studies report in The Lancet. And there are no signs of slowing down, the researchers write in a commentary about the studies." [33]

Make sure you refer and document your C-section preferences in your Birth Plan.

****

CHAPTER 8
Birth Plan

A birth plan is critical to develop early on in your pregnancy, as it accomplishes several things. It will help you make crucial decisions concerning what you envision and request the birth to look like. It can help guide you through the research and discernment process, and give you a framework to share with your birth "team." It helps eliminate any confusion for all parties involved and gives parents a sense of security and empowerment. Below is a sample birth plan if you don't know where to start. You can add, revise, or eliminate the items included to make it personal for you and your family.

Be sure to read through this entire sample birth plan as there are several other recommendations included related to the birth process not discussed up to this point in this book.

Sample Birth Plan – BEFORE Labor Begins

- My practitioner will seek my opinion concerning all issues directly affecting my baby's birth before deviating from my Birth Plan.
- I would like to labor at home as long as possible.
- If Fetal Non-Stress Test (NST) observation is recommended after my due date, I am flexible and support this procedure.
- If all is well with baby and I and it is less than 14 days past my "due date," I prefer to go into labor naturally rather than be induced.
- I do not want to have "Artificial Rupture" or "Stripping of Membranes" (the doctor or midwife will sweep a gloved finger between the membranes of the amniotic sac in your uterus in the efforts of speeding up your labor).
- If my water breaks before I go into labor, I would like to wait 48 hours before being induced.
- If birthing equipment is available, I would like to use a (choose to include all that apply): Birthing bed, birthing ball, bean bag chair, birthing tub/pool/shower, birthing stool, and/or squatting bar.

Environmental Settings – select all that apply:

I request:
- To have dimmed lights.
- People entering the room to speak softly.
- No one speak during the delivery.
- To wear my own clothes during labor and delivery.
- To have a TV/radio/CD player available for my pre-selected music.
- To wear headsets during my labor and delivery.
- To have my birth photographed.
- To have my birth filmed/videotaped.
- To wear my glasses or contact lenses unless removal becomes medically necessary.

First Stage Labor

I request:
- Not to be separated from _____ at any point during labor or birth.
- To limit internal exams unless they are absolutely necessary and agreed upon by all parties.
- To avoid a catheter; please allow me to walk to the bathroom to empty my bladder.
- To not be connected to an IV. If an emergency arises, it would be acceptable at that time.
- Not to use any monitoring devices throughout labor. I agree to have them attached if an emergency arises, or for a maximum of 2-5 minutes every hour.
- Not to be offered drugs for the management of pain. If an emergency arises, we would like to be informed of our options prior to the administration of any drug or procedure, and what the possible side effects of our decision would be.
- Flexibility determining the best possible positions for my comfort during delivery with the freedom to walk and ability to change positions as desired.

Second Stage Labor

I request:

- To risk a tear, rather than have an episiotomy. If possible, use counter pressure to avoid tearing.
- To try any position that feels right to me at the time of delivery
- Avoiding a Cesarean unless absolutely crucial. If deemed medically necessary, _____ should be present at all times during surgery.
- To labor my baby down, and not be instructed to push. I would like to wait for my natural urge to push.
- To not allow any devices such as vacuum extraction or forceps to be used during the delivery.

Third Stage Labor

I request:

- My baby be placed on my abdomen immediately to begin bonding and breastfeeding as soon as possible.
- To save our baby's umbilical cord blood. Some parents choose to do this because "Umbilical cord blood stem cells can be used in transplants to treat a variety of pediatric disorders including leukemia, sickle cell disease, and metabolic disorders. Patients who need a cord blood transplant can currently try to find a match with a sibling or from an unrelated person. An autologous (self) transplant can also be done if a child's umbilical cord blood has been stored in a private cord blood bank." [34] This private use storage has costs associated with it but you can also choose to donate it to a public bank at no charge (see appendix).
- The placenta to be delivered naturally, allowing full time for expulsion without any medication or physical assistance, specifically, no pulling or holding the umbilical cord taut.
- Not to have the baby bathed at all. We wish to leave the vernix (white, waxy substance covering the baby's body) to be absorbed naturally or even rubbed in to the baby's skin.
- All newborn procedures to take place in our presence. If I am unable to be with the baby for newborn procedures, I would like _____ to stay with the baby at all times.

- 24-hour rooming-in as there is no need for our baby stay in the nursery.
- Not to circumcise our baby if a male at this time.
- Not to vaccinate as we are choosing to wait at this time.

To breastfeed exclusively. Please do not introduce any pacifiers, baby bottles, or nipples of any type.

Save the placenta. If you are considering saving your placenta to consume later, research your options as to how it will be preserved before you go into labor. As the placenta is an organ, it is full of nutrients, vitamins, and minerals. These include iron, prolactin (used to produce breast milk), prostaglandin (helps contract the uterus after giving birth), and oxytocin (the hormone that helps with bonding). There are companies that will dehydrate and encapsulate your placenta for you as well.

We respect the professional judgment of the doctors and will of course be flexible in the event of complications. Although we feel confident everything will progress in a normal fashion, we have confidence you will inform us immediately if any problems arise. This will allow us to discuss available alternatives and make responsible decisions. We appreciate your attention to our birth preferences and are grateful for the kind and encouraging care you provide.

****

CHAPTER 9
Postpartum Considerations for Mom

You have made it this far in the process which is a great accomplishment! Many mothers and fathers get to the other end of the birth process and are instantly overwhelmed. The joy is like nothing else they have ever experienced and the enormous responsibility of becoming a parent quickly sets in. Hopefully, the suggestions in this section have been on the radar before now so the stress levels remain low.

Breastfeeding

First, it is critical I point out breastfeeding will always be best for your baby, and ideally for a minimum of 12 to 18 months. According to the World Health Organization, "Breastfeeding is an unequalled way of providing ideal food for the healthy growth and development of infants; it is also an integral part of the reproductive process with important implications for the health of mothers. As a global public health recommendation, infants should be exclusively breastfed for the first six months of life to achieve optimal growth, development, and health. After that, to meet their evolving nutritional requirements, infants should receive nutritionally adequate and safe complementary foods while breastfeeding continues for up to two years of age or beyond. Exclusive breastfeeding from birth is possible except for a few medical conditions, and unrestricted exclusive breastfeeding results in ample milk production." [35]

"The World Health Organization (WHO) and the American Academy of Pediatrics (AAP) emphasize the value of breastfeeding for mothers as well as children. Both recommend exclusive breastfeeding for the first six months of life. The AAP recommends that supplemented breastfeeding follow this for at least one year, while WHO recommends that supplemented breastfeeding continue up to two years or more." [36]

There are several good pumps on the market, so if away from home, you can pump breast milk and freeze for future use.

When I was working full time while breastfeeding my first. I traveled quite a bit, so it was more challenging, but I was able to make it work. I would take my pump to work and my employer was kind enough to add a lock to one of the conference room doors for me. I would collect breast milk and store it in the employee freezer. One time, I was traveling for 5 days and my husband was running out of the supply we had at home. So, I collected the milk on my trip and flew it back home, my husband meeting the plane at the airport – crisis averted!

Our story was even featured in a 2004 article:

"Sending home a unique care package –

Kimberly Roberto's job as an E-commerce Operations Manager for GE Supply had her out of town up to three times a month. Her husband traveled several times a year to chiropractic conventions. How did their travel affect the childcare scenario? 'Mostly, we would just buckle down and ask favors from family.'

When business brought her near her parents Connecticut home, she brought her young son along, leaving grandma and grandpa on babysitting duty. 'I didn't feel guilty leaving him home without me again.'

When her oldest son was six months old, the now mother of three had to travel to Dallas, TX for a five-day training session. Determined to continue breastfeeding, she brought her breast pump and stocked the milk in a freezer provided by the hotel. 'Imagine trying to find places to pump while traveling to different locations. You name it, I pumped there: my rental car, storage closets, bathrooms, back offices, etc. It was interesting to say the least.'

As anticipated, her husband ran out of breast milk at home. So she gathered up all the bags she had stored up during the trip, packed them in ice, and marched to the airport. 'I sent my precious package via Delta Dash back to Atlanta.' She said. 'My liquid gold had its own flight back home where my husband had to go pick it up. It was comical, but sweet!'

Inability to Breastfeed or Low Milk Production

I would encourage you to exhaust all attempts to naturally remedy the situation first. However, if breastfeeding isn't an option due to health concerns, extremely low milk production, medications you do not wish transferred to the baby, adoption, or twins, one is able to source another woman's breast milk. There are breast milk "banks" and social media sites which match mothers together for donated breast milk. Of course, you want to investigate the mother's lifestyle habits and how the breast milk is collected and stored, but it is a second-best option.

Another option would be to make your own homemade formula. There are some other premade formulas that are a good option if none of the others work.

In case of low milk production, you might try these techniques in order to attempt increasing your milk supply:

- Schedule an adjustment
- Ensure hydration
- Crawl into bed with your baby
- Relax!

Fenugreek tea, blessed thistle tea, and lfalfa/fennel tea have been known to increase milk production. However, as with any regiment change, always check first with your Holistic Care Provider to ensure you do not have potential contraindications with these herbs.

Your Diet While Breastfeeding

You are still eating for two since the quality of your breast milk depends largely on what you are eating. You will quickly discover you will need to eat more than you typically do. Focus on healthy whole foods. You should be maintaining a high intake of omega 3's to help your baby's developing immune system. Lacto-fermented foods such as sauerkraut, kimchi (careful – spiciness could be an issue), kefir, and kombucha are also especially helpful. Avoid caffeine, alcohol, and soy products. It is advisable with the consultation of your physician to supplement with prenatal nutraceuticals.

Great Nutraceutical Considerations to Consult With Your Physician

I highly recommend MaxLiving Prenatal Daily Essentials Packets.

Postpartum Exercise

It is imperative to take your time easing back into exercising after giving birth. Your body has been through an extensive ordeal and it is especially important to attend to your entire pelvic floor, allowing it to properly heal. It is also important to avoid injury, incorporating functional movements as you will be carrying around increased weight. Consider all the increased movements your body will experience: bending over and picking up your baby, carrying around heavy diaper bags, lugging the car seat between vehicles, and all those other interactions with your newly-purchased baby gear. Once past the first two phases of post-partum, I recommend the maxT3 program (see appendix), and consulting with your MaxLiving Doctor and staff for specific recommendations regarding exercise post-pregnancy (see appendix). Typically post-partum is considered in three phases: Phase 1 is 6-12 hours, Phase 2 is 2-6 weeks, and Phase 3 is up to 6 months.

Chiropractic

Postpartum chiropractic care is absolutely crucial and necessary immediately after birth through the duration of breastfeeding. Although lifetime chiropractic care should be a priority, it certainly is essential during the postpartum period. The entire pregnancy, labor and delivery process can be very taxing on the neurological and biomechanical systems, and there will be continual changes to your body following birth. For example, the ligaments will begin to tighten up as hormones like Estrogen and Relaxin begin to return back to their normal levels. It is imperative the spine and pelvis be adjusted back to normal positions as these ligaments begin to tighten. Otherwise, the mechanical but natural insult occurring during the pregnancy can result in a lifetime of issues.

Antidepressants and Birth Defects

Many women deal with anxiety and depression before and during pregnancy, and are concerned they will experience postpartum depression after the delivery. Consider discussing your apprehensions with your MaxLiving Doctor or Primary Holistic Health Care Physician. However, it is important to understand the risks of taking a prescribed anti-depressant while pregnant.

A Study in the Canadian Medical Association Journal reported a 68% increase in miscarriages in women who take antidepressants.[37]

Paxil increases the risk by 75%. In 2010, Glaxo Smith Kline entered into a confidential settlement with nearly 200 families who claim Paxil caused congenital birth defects[38] "Effexor, Lexapro, Celexa, Prozac and Zoloft during the first trimester of their pregnancy were significantly more likely to miscarry than women who did not take antidepressants. Researchers found that the risk associated with miscarriage was 68 percent higher in women who used the drugs. The researchers also found that Effexor was among the antidepressants which carried the highest risk." [39]

In October 2009, a Philadelphia jury awarded Lyam Kilker's family $2.5 million in compensatory damages after he was born with three cardiac defects after his mother was prescribed Paxil.[40, 41]

Vaccine Information

This is a highly-charged topic, and there is a plethora of information readily available about the pros of vaccination, but the cons are discussed with far less frequency. It is my intention to provide accurate and relevant information for informed decisions to be made. Keep an open mind and do your own research.

Research indicates:

Vaccines are not the reason for a decline in the incidence of disease. Significant improvements in hygiene and sanitation, such as the introduction of refrigeration, water filtration, and workplace safety, are to thank for decreased disease rates.[42]

Regardless of what you might hear, no vaccine offers genuine 100% immunity. Vaccinated individuals are often more susceptible to disease.[43]

Almost all vaccines contain toxic contaminants like mercury, formaldehyde, MSG, antibiotics, squalene, Polysorbate 80, and shockingly, even aborted fetal tissue. These toxins can produce dangerous side effects and reactions ranging from soreness, reduced immune function, brain damage, and even death. Many symptoms from effects are not observed until years after the vaccination, and no one really knows the long-term effects of vaccines. We now have a whole nation of people with lowered immune responses and the typical S.A.D. (Standard American Diet) further depleting it. We also have witnessed a drastic rise in autism, auto-immune disorders, learning disorders, and ADHD. As discussed earlier in the chapter "Prenatal Considerations," people who possess the genetic "MTHFR" SNP need to research this far more diligently as introducing any type of toxin, especially vaccinations with this genetic SNP, can wreck-havoc if not approached carefully and cautiously.[44, 45]

The development and marketing of vaccines is surrounded by conflicts of interest. Many scientists involved with the vaccine governing bodies in the CDC are on pharmaceutical payrolls, own lucrative pharmaceutical stocks, and some even have patents on the vaccines they are mandating.[46,47]

Our bodies were created with an amazing ability to heal, provided there is no interference. Whether it is dirt, dust, dander, viruses, or bacteria, every irritant is a necessary challenge to be overcome by our innate immune system. As exercise is helpful to the muscles, the immune system grows stronger with every natural challenge it encounters (germs, bacteria, etc.).

A MaxLiving lifestyle, characterized by a healthy nervous system, a whole food based anti-inflammatory diet, a strong fit body, and a peaceful, purpose-filled life is what you were created for. You are equipped with the keys for excellent health. So please, educate yourself before you vaccinate.

****

CHAPTER 10
Postpartum Considerations for Baby

Your baby's first adjustment

The birth process is physically taxing for mom and baby. Many of the very first subluxations (misalignments) in a child result from the labor process. It is extremely important to have your baby checked by a chiropractor as soon as possible after birth. The doctors will gladly come to your home, birth center, or hospital. This can drastically reduce the worsening of subluxations which many times results in other health consequences.

Additional support for chiropractic care in children:

While there is much research available, I am highlighting just a few here.

- **Tonsillitis:** Lewit found among primarily youthful patients with chronic tonsillitis, 92% had an atlanto-occipital (C1-C2 Vertebrae) blockage. After correction of the blockage, recurrence was absent, no tonsillectomy was required. [48]

- **Scoliosis:** Siefert found among 1,093 newborns, 298 children with atlanto-occipital blockages significantly connected with the development of a C-scoliosis.

- **Blocked Nerve Impulses:** Blocked nerve impulses at the atlas (C1) may cause many clinical features ranging from central motor impairment to lower infection resistance – especially ear nose and throat infections. Gutmann and other German medical studies concluded that approximately 80% of all children are not in autonomic balance and that many experience atlas blockage or subluxation.[49] Out of 211 five-day-old babies suffering from vomiting hyperactivity and sleeplessness, 95% revealed cervical strain. Specific correction of the strain frequently resulted in immediate quieting, cessation of crying, muscular relaxation, & sleepiness. [50]

- **Sudden Infant Death Syndrome:** Dr. Abraham Towbin, a Harvard researcher, found that spinal injury from the birth process was responsible for SIDS in 7 out of 8 autopsies. [51]

- (Towbin A: Latent Spinal Cord and Brain Stem Injury in Newborn Infants. Develop Med Child Nerol. 1969 Feb: 11 (1): 54-68)

Colic – According to a 2013 Study published in the Journal of Clinical Chiropractic Pediatrics, "The current study revealed that excessively crying infants were 5 times less likely to cry significantly, if they were treated with chiropractic manual therapy, and that chiropractic care reduced their crying times by about 50%, compared with those infants provided solely medical management." [52]

Ear Infections – Ear infections are extremely commonplace but they are not normal. The smallest bones in the body are located in our ears. After the trauma of passing through the birth canal, these bones can misalign, creating the perfect environment for ear infections to develop in your baby.

"If a child has had a fall, for example, and has caused a minor misalignment in one of the vertebrae in the neck, the irritation caused by that problem is sufficient to cause the neck muscles to develop a state of increased tension or spasm. The resulting muscle contraction, especially in the area of the sternocleidomastoid muscle (SCM), can be the cause of restricted lymph drainage from the ear." [53]

Circumcision

Circumcision is not necessary for health reasons. However, many people choose circumcision for social and religious reasons. If you do decide to circumcise your baby boy, it is best to wait eight days. This time frame allows the baby's blood to clot better and provides time for him to learn how to breastfeed first and associate with being comforted. Insist either you or your spouse be present during the procedure, understanding it will hurt, resulting in considerable pain and crying. Mom should be nearby to offer her breast for this immediate comfort. Be sure to care for the cut afterward by closely following your doctor's instructions. Avoid any petroleum products like Vaseline and consider coconut oil as a natural alternative instead.

Bouncers, Baby Carriers

Never use any product or device that allows your baby to sit in an upright position before 6 months of age. A baby's spine is not yet fully developed and downward pressure can impact the development of the proper curves of the spine.

Introducing Solid Food to Babies

Once your baby's pearly whites start to come in, it is an indication they are almost ready for solid food. Contrary to typical health advice, "conventional" commercial dairy is not desirable. If you decide to introduce dairy, wait at least 12 months, introducing organic cow's milk or organic goat's milk. Goat's milk is much easier to digest as the protein molecule is much smaller than those in cow's milk.

When introducing foods, do so one at a time and see how your baby reacts to each new introduction. Always wait at least four days before introducing the next food, as this helps detect any food sensitivities or allergic reactions.

Where to Start

Always buy organic when possible.

Starting with vegetables is ideal. A few great food items to begin with are avocados, sweet potatoes, squash, and green beans.

Serve the pureed vegetables with organic butter to help assimilate the nutrient content.

Introducing sweet foods like fruit early on sets the child up for a "sweet tooth" later in life. After your baby is accustomed to the above foods, you can introduce some fruits, such as apples, peaches, pears, and plums.

Always start new foods slightly cooked (steaming is preferable), then move to raw. When baby is about nine months old you can start adding more vegetables to the child's diet such as broccoli, cauliflower, zucchini, asparagus, spinach, etc. Tomatoes are technically a fruit, but are great addition too.

An excellent food for your growing baby is egg yolk. These little encapsulated punches of protein contain healthy omega-3's, amino acids, and the ever-valuable cholesterol necessary for nourishing brain development. This good cholesterol is not, nor has it ever been, the enemy, contrary to what you were taught in school. Thankfully that "opinion" changed in recent years and eggs finally came back in the good graces of our government. The whites of the egg are usually easier to digest after a baby reaches the age of 12 to 18 months. The best way to prepare egg yolks for your baby is to boil a free-range egg for 3 1/2 minutes, then peel the shell, removing the egg white for anyone else to enjoy. The yolk should be soft and warm, but not too hot as heat will break down enzymes.

Around 12 months of age, if you have decided on and would like to add grains to the baby's diet, this would be the appropriate time. Only purchase organic, healthy whole grains like brown rice, sprouted grains, quinoa, millet, or oatmeal (from a gluten free facility). Many parents are tempted to add cereals in early, which can lead to undesired consequences. Adding grains too soon can lead to obesity, overeating, food allergies, and hormonal imbalances. Never add cereals to a bottle as a baby's sucking and swallowing coordination is not yet fully developed. Besides, their digestive system is much better suited to digest fat and proteins rather than carbohydrates from grains.

Lastly, at 12 to 18 months of age, you can add organic meats, eggs, and nuts/seeds (preferably soaked for easier digestion). It is not recommended, but if you stop breastfeeding before 12 months, consider adding organic, naturally-raised meats sooner than if you would continue breastfeeding.

Preparing Baby Food

Making your own baby food is quick, easy, and much healthier for baby than conventional baby foods as you simply steam vegetables. It is ideal to make enough vegetables for the older children/adults in the house to eat, and use the extra to prepare for your baby. Transfer the steamed vegetables to a blender or food processor, add a pat or two of organic butter, and process until pureed. Add a bit of filtered water if need be for desired consistency.

Storing Baby Food

Transfer the pureed food to glass jars for storing in the refrigerator. Another suggestion for longer storage: transfer the food to non-toxic ice cube trays or other small storage containers to freeze. Then, just pop food cubes out as needed.

****

Conclusion

This book contains so much good and vital information for this exciting stage of your life, and I am so thankful you are now armed with real knowledge. It is essential to have solid resources at your fingertips to make informed decisions on your health prior to and during pregnancy, birth, delivery, and beyond. I encourage you to visit and discuss any issues that may arise with your MaxLiving Doctor.

Keep learning! Continue research on your own, embracing the amazing gift you have been blessed with as mother and father. It is a time of your life you will never forget and you will wish to create the best memories possible. Be confident in yourself and the fact God designed your body perfectly for this transformation and transference of life.

Kimberly & Dr. Fred Roberto

Recipes

Breakfast
Smoothies & Beverages
Soups
Salads & Slaws
Entrées
Sides & Appetizers
Desserts

 Core Plan   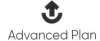 Advanced Plan   Vegan   Vegetarian

Breakfast

Smoked Salmon Hash
Chia & Almond Milk Pudding
Mini Onion Quiches

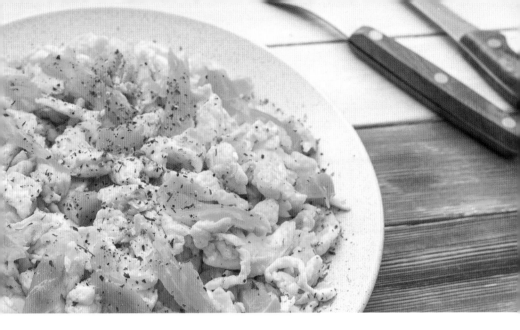

Smoked Salmon Hash

 COURSE
Breakfast

 CUISINE
American

 1 SERVING

 COOK TIME
5 minutes

This advanced plan meal will leave you wanting to make it again! The wild-caught smoked salmon and free range eggs help make this a yummy and nutritious meal!

INGREDIENTS

- 2 organic eggs, free range, scrambled
- ½–¾ cup smoked salmon, chopped into small bits
- 1-2 tbsp organic cream cheese
- fresh or dried dill to taste
- sea salt and pepper to taste
- 1 tbsp coconut oil or butter

Optional
- additional herbs and spices
- spinach
- kale
- diced onions

INSTRUCTIONS

1. Heat a non-toxic skillet on the stove.
2. Add butter or coconut oil and heat until melted.
3. Add eggs and cook until stiffened but not completely done.
4. Add the rest of the ingredients and mix well. Serve immediately.

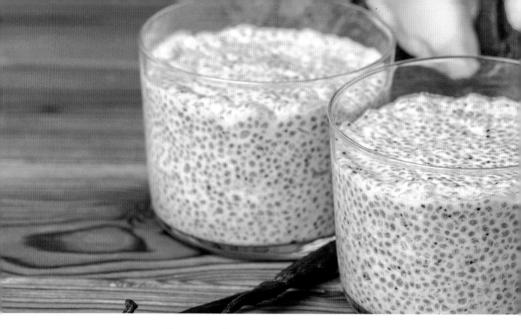

Chia & Almond Milk Pudding
Raw & Healthy

 COURSE
Breakfast

 CUISINE
American

 3 SERVINGS

 COOK TIME
1 hour

Chia seeds are a power food high in fiber, calcium, antioxidants, and omega-3 fatty acids, making them a great protein-packed addition to your diet! When mixed with liquid, they plump, giving the mixture a tapioca-like consistency. Get all of the benefits of chia seeds with this tasty chia seed pudding! This raw recipe takes just a few minutes to make and its protein and nutrient content it the perfect quick, on-the-go breakfast. This recipe is extremely versatile as well — top it with your favorite fruits, nuts, seeds, or coconut.

INGREDIENTS

- ¾ cup chia seeds
- 4 cups almond milk
- 2 vanilla beans (split down the center and seeds removed) *(or 2 tsps vanilla extract)*
- 6-8 tbsp erythritol *(like Swerve or stevia, to taste)*

INSTRUCTIONS

1. Add almond milk, vanilla, and sweetener to a blender and mix well.
2. With the blender on a very low setting, add the chia seeds and mix. If you would like to add other ingredients, do it here.
3. Transfer to a container and stir every 5 minutes for the first 15 minutes, then let sit for 30 minutes to 1 hour. Transfer to the refrigerator.
4. When ready to serve, add toppings.

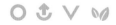

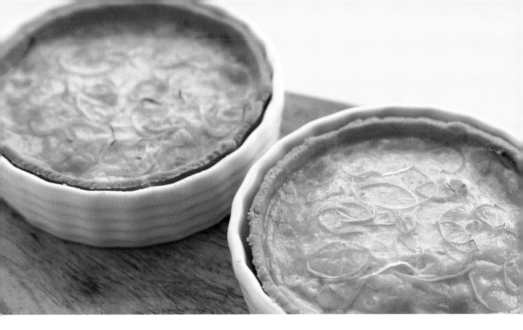

Mini Onion Quiches

 COURSE
Breakfast

 CUISINE
American

 6 SERVINGS

 COOK TIME
30 minutes

These mini quiches are great to freeze for a quick on the go breakfast later. Here, a typical crust is substituted with shredded coconut.

INGREDIENTS

- ¾ cup shredded coconut
- 4 tbsp butter, melted (for crust)
- 1 cup chopped green onion with tops
- 2 tbsp butter (for onions)
- 2 eggs
- 1 cup whole milk, grass-fed
- ½ tsp sea salt
- ¼ tsp pepper
- 1 cup swiss cheese, grated

INSTRUCTIONS

1. Preheat oven to 300°F.
2. Combine coconut and melted butter.
3. Divide coconut among mini muffin tins.
4. Sauté onion for 10 minutes in 2 tablespoons butter.
5. Cool onions, then divide evenly over coconut crust.
6. Beat eggs, add milk, salt, pepper, and swiss cheese.
7. Pour by spoonfuls on top of onions in tins.
8. Do not fill to the top as they will run over.
9. Bake until set, about 15-20 minutes.

Do Not Overbake.

Smoothies

Max Fitterade
Avocado & Spinach Smoothie
Pistachio Ice Cream/Smoothie
Very Berry Smoothie

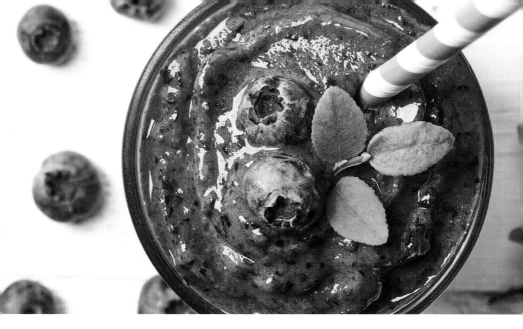

Max Fitterade

| COURSE
Drinks | CUISINE
American | 1 SERVING | COOK TIME
5 minutes |

This is a great way to replenish electrolytes lost during a workout since it uses coconut water. It is super-hydrating and has the added benefit of high-antioxidant berries.

INGREDIENTS

- 8 oz coconut water, preferably raw
- ½–1 cup frozen berries (if using fresh, add ¼ cup ice)
- ½–1 juice of lemon to taste
- dash liquid stevia, if desired

INSTRUCTIONS

1. Blend everything in a high-powered blender or Vitamix.
2. Enjoy!

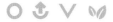

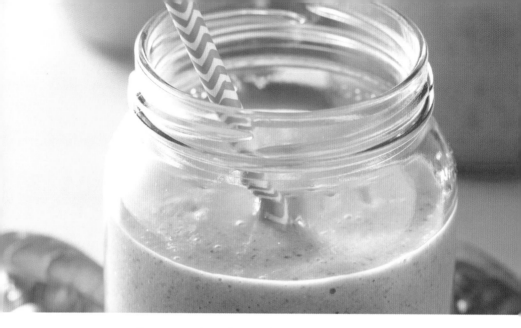

Avocado & Spinach Smoothie
Healthy Green Shake

 COURSE
Breakfast,
Drinks

 CUISINE
American

 1 SERVING

 COOK TIME
5 minutes

Naturally green and ultra-creamy, this avocado and spinach smoothie is sure to be your family's year-round favorite. This healthy green shake features peppermint oil for a delicious minty twist. For an extra treat, blend in some cacao nibs. Healthy green smoothies have never tasted better!

INGREDIENTS

- 1 organic avocado
- 1½ cups ice
- 1 cup organic spinach
- 1-3 drops peppermint oil/extract (make sure to use an oil/extract made for ingestion)
- Stevia (to taste)
- optional: cacao nibs (to taste)
- water/almond milk (as needed)

INSTRUCTIONS

1. Add all ingredients (except water/almond milk) to blender and mix until smooth.
2. Add additional liquid such as water or almond milk, as needed, to allow for easier blending.
3. Serve chilled in a glass with or without ice.

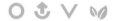

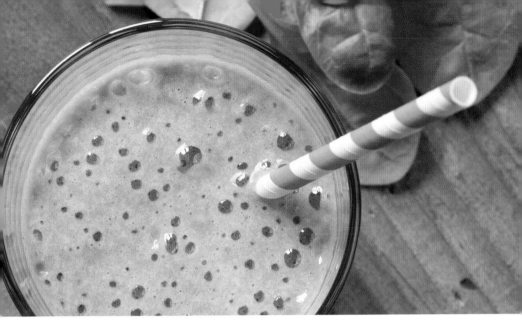

Pistachio Ice Cream/Smoothie

 COURSE
Drinks

 CUISINE
American

 2 SERVINGS

 COOK TIME
5 minutes

This recipe was inspired by a pistachio ice cream smoothie maker demonstration. This has been adapted to use core plan approved ingredients, and has added protein for extra nutritional value. You won't believe how delicious this is!

INGREDIENTS

- 1 ½ cup coconut milk, full-fat
- ½ cup organic spinach (or more)
- ⅔ cup shelled pistachios
- ½ avocado
- 2-3 scoop Grass-Fed Whey Protein Chocolate or Vanilla
- 2 cups ice
- more stevia to taste

INSTRUCTIONS

1. Blend everything together using the plunger.
2. This can be eaten with a straw or spoon, with a pistachio garnish.

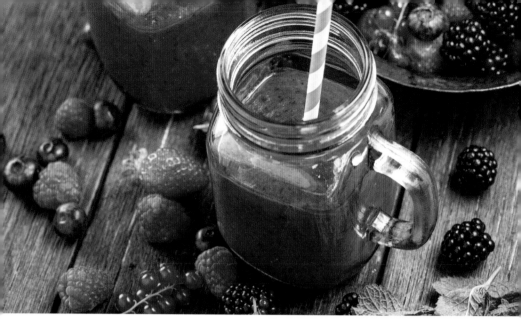

Very Berry Smoothie
Easy & Healthy Smoothies

 COURSE
Drinks

 CUISINE
American

 2 SERVINGS

 COOK TIME
5 minutes

This delicious, healthy smoothie is filled with all of your favorite berries. With the addition of protein powder, this berry smoothie is a great option to start your day, drink after a workout, or when you're craving something sweet!

INGREDIENTS

- 1 large handful of berries (any mixture of strawberries, blueberries, blackberries, or raspberries)
- ½ cup coconut milk, almond milk, organic milk, or organic plain yogurt
- ¼ cup filtered water (have additional water for consistency changes)
- 1 scoop Grass-Fed Whey Protein (vanilla)

INSTRUCTIONS

1. Put all ingredients in a heavy-duty blender and blend to desired consistency.
2. You may add additional water if necessary.

Soups

Easy Tex-Mex Soup
Homemade Chicken Soup
White Turkey Chili
Chicken Soup With Broccoli,
Spinach, and Cauliflower
Super Veggie Minestrone Soup

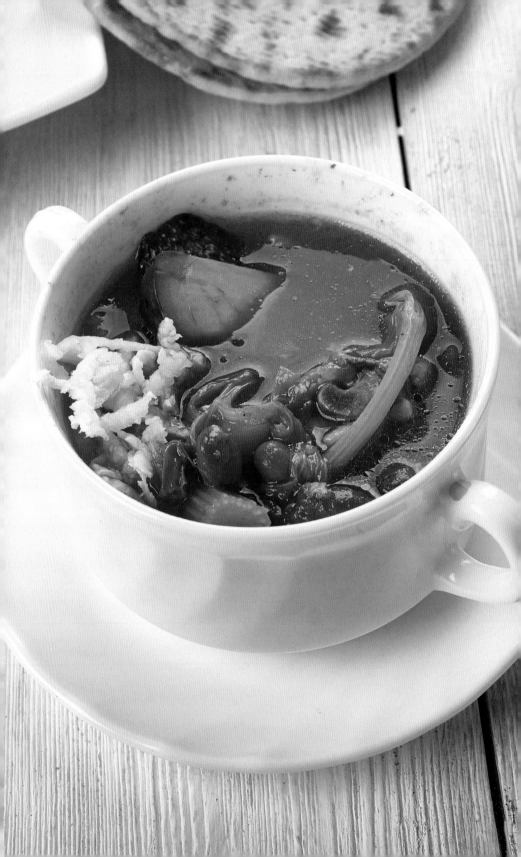

Easy Tex-Mex Soup

 COURSE
Soup

 CUISINE
Tex-Mex

6 SERVINGS

COOK TIME
15 minutes

This is a great go-to dish that is so flexible and easy to make. You can pretty much use any veggies you have on hand and spice it up however you please. Don't limit yourself to just the ingredients listed below. Mix it up and have fun!

INGREDIENTS

- 4 cup organic free-range chicken broth
- 1 roma tomato (or ½ regular tomato)
- 1 rib organic celery
- 1 carrot (core plan only)
- 1 onion, sliced
- 1 clove garlic
- ½ organic red yellow or orange bell pepper
- small slice of cabbage green, savoy, napa
- 1-2 mushrooms
- handful of organic yellow squash or zucchini
- 1 tsp chili powder
- sea salt and pepper to taste

- ⅛ tsp cumin
- ½ fresh jalapeno pepper (add more for a spicier taste)
- ½ cup organic cooked chicken
- ¼ cup black olives
- handful organic non-GMO corn (core plan only)
- 1 organic sprouted grain tortilla found in the frozen section of health food stores, (core plan only)

Garnish: avocados, cilantro, organic sour cream

INSTRUCTIONS

1. Using a high-powered blender, place all ingredients except chicken, olives, corn (core plan only), and tortillas (core plan only) and blend on high until everything is liquified.
2. Turn off blender and add chicken, jalapenos, olives, corn, and tortilla (torn into pieces).
3. Put your blender on low speed and blend for 10-20 seconds. You will want the last batch of ingredients to remain in small chunks.
4. Transfer to a saucepan and heat.

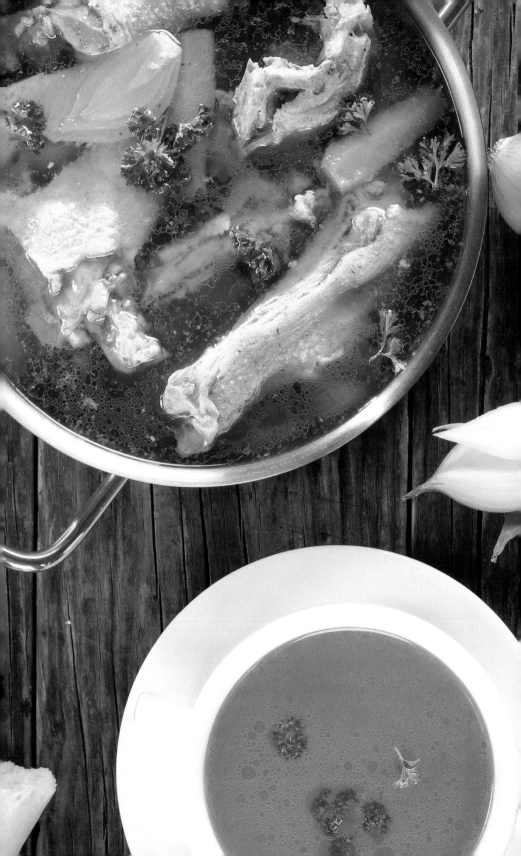

Homemade Chicken Soup

 COURSE
Soup

 CUISINE
American

8 SERVINGS

 COOK TIME
3 hours

This is the good old fashioned way of making chicken soup. The kind your grandmother used to make. The taste is so different than the chicken soup most Americans are used to eating, that people think there is some sort of magic formula. It is really very simple. Soup out of a can or made from bouillon cubes is not real chicken soup and it is certainly not healthy. Most commercial soups are loaded with table salt, MSG, and other flavorings and additives, but not this homemade delight.

INGREDIENTS

- 1 whole free-range, organic chicken
- 6-8 qt filtered water
- 1 bunch celery with tops (~5 stalks)
- 12 carrots
- 1 whole onion
- 1 bunch parsley, stems included
- 4 tbsp sea salt
- 3 tbsp black pepper

INSTRUCTIONS

1. Place the chicken in a large stockpot and fill with filtered water.
2. Wash the celery and six of the carrots, cut in half. Cut the onion into quarters. Wash the parsley. Add everything to the pot and bring to a boil.
3. Boil everything for about 2-3 hours, skimming the foam that rises to the top periodically.
4. Put a colander over another large stock pot and pour the soup through the colander retaining only the broth. Put the broth back on the stove and simmer.
5. Let the chicken cool until it able to be handled.
6. Carefully take all of the meat off of the bones and add it back to the stockpot. You can have the chunks of chicken as big or as small as you want. You can also start skimming off some of the fat that rises to the top.
7. Add sea salt and pepper to the pot because you are not using any bouillon you will need to add quite a bit of salt. Just keep tasting it).
8. If you need more broth, you can add in a couple of containers of organic, free range chicken broth (check ingredients).
9. Chop the remaining 6 carrots and 5 celery stalks and add them to the pot. Simmer until vegetables are soft. Refrigerate the soup overnight.
10. In the morning, you will be able to skim off the fat that solidifies on the surface.
11. Reheat the soup when ready to eat and add whole wheat noodles if desired. ENJOY!

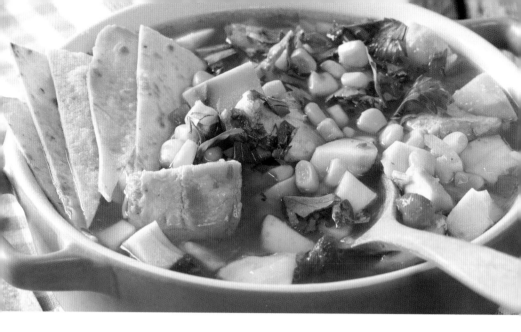

White Turkey Chili

 COURSE
Soup

 CUISINE
American, Tex-Mex

 6 SERVINGS

 COOK TIME
45 minutes

This is a great alternative to red chili. It is great as leftovers and easily packed in a thermos for transport.

INGREDIENTS

- 1 tbsp olive oil
- 1 medium onion, diced
- 2 stalks celery, diced
- 3 medium poblano peppers, seeded and white ribs removed, finely diced
- 1 clove garlic, minced
- 1 tsp ground cumin
- ½ tsp ground coriander
- ¼ tsp cayenne pepper or more if you like it spicy
- 2 lb ground white meat turkey
- 30 oz white beans such as cannellini, drained and rinsed
- 8 cup organic free-range chicken broth
- ¾ tsp dried oregano
- sea salt
- 2 tbsp fresh cilantro leaves, chopped, optional
- 1 avocado chopped, optional

INSTRUCTIONS

1. Heat the oil in large pot or Dutch oven over moderate heat.
2. Add the onion, celery, and peppers, and cook, stirring occasionally, until the vegetables are soft, about 8 minutes.
3. Add the garlic, cumin, coriander and cayenne and cook, stirring about 30 seconds.
4. Add the ground turkey and cook, breaking up the meat with a spoon, until the meat is no longer pink about 2 minutes.
5. Add the white beans, broth and oregano. Cook, partially covered, stirring occasionally, for 25 minutes.
6. Add the salt and more cayenne pepper, to taste, and continue cooking, partially covered, 10 minutes longer.
7. Ladle into individual bowls and top with cilantro and garnish with avocados if desired.

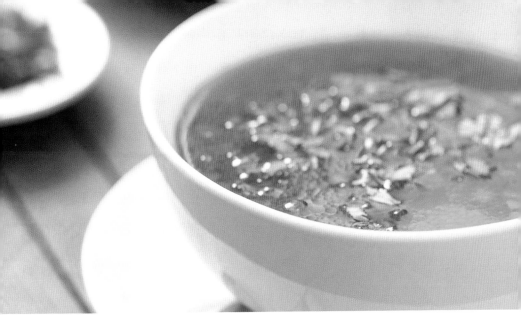

Chicken Soup With Broccoli, Spinach, and Cauliflower

 COURSE
Soup

 CUISINE
American

 4 SERVINGS

 COOK TIME
30 minutes

Try our delicious chicken soup recipe full of nutrients. A classy, keto-friendly alternative to regular chicken and vegetable soup, with a healthy, tasty twist!

INGREDIENTS

- 6 cups organic chicken broth (use bone broth for extra nutrients)
- 1 cage-free chicken breast, skinless and boneless
- 1 yellow onion, finely-diced
- ½ cup broccoli florets
- ½ cup cauliflower florets
- ½ cup chopped spinach
- 3 tbsp finely-chopped fresh parsley
- sea salt (to taste)
- fresh ground pepper (to taste)

INSTRUCTIONS

1. In a large sauce pan, bring chicken broth to a simmer.
2. Add the chicken breast and simmer just until tender and no trace of pink remains, (about 8-10 minutes).
3. Remove the chicken breast. Transfer to a cutting board and cut into 1-inch cubes. Set aside.
4. Add the onions, broccoli, cauliflower, and chopped spinach to the broth. Simmer for 10 minutes.
5. Add the cubed chicken, parsley, sea salt, and pepper.
6. Simmer 3 more minutes.
7. Ladle out a serving, garnish and enjoy!

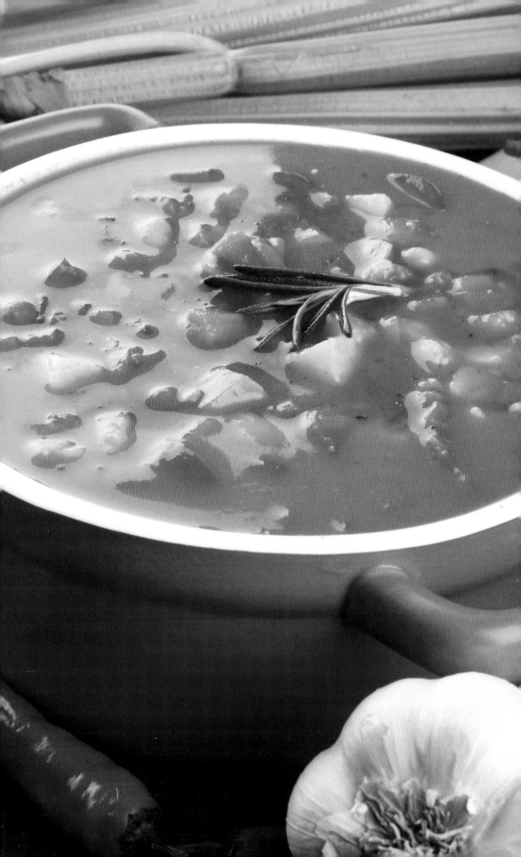

Super Veggie Minestrone Soup

 COURSE
Soup

 CUISINE
Italian

 4 SERVINGS

COOK TIME
1 hour

This yummy veggie packed soup is perfect for a cool night or reheated for a quick lunch! Try it out today, and you'll be happy you did!

INGREDIENTS

- 2 tsp coconut oil
- 1 medium yellow onion
- 2 tsp fresh oregano, chopped, or ½ teaspoon dried oregano
- 2 tsp minced garlic
- 2 medium organic yellow squash, chopped
- 2 medium organic zucchini, chopped
- 2 medium carrots, chopped
- 6 organic Roma tomatoes, chopped
- 40 oz. free range chicken broth, divided

- 1 can great northern beans, rinsed & drained
- 6 oz. bag of fresh baby spinach or 5-6 leaves kale stems, removed and chopped
- ¾ tsp sea salt
- ¼ tsp freshly ground black pepper
- 1 cup grated asiago or parmesan cheese

INSTRUCTIONS

1. Heat oil in a dutch oven over medium high heat.
2. Add onion to pan and sauté until softened, stirring frequently. Add oregano, garlic, sea salt, and pepper and heat through.
3. Stir in squash, zucchini, and carrot sauté about 5 more minutes or until vegetables are tender.
4. While the vegetables are cooking, place all but one cup of the chopped Roma tomatoes and a small amount of the broth in a blender and blend to a smooth consistency.
5. Add the tomato mixture along with the remaining chopped tomatoes, beans, and the remaining broth. If using kale, add it here.
6. Bring to a boil, then reduce heat; simmer about 20 minutes.
7. Remove from heat. If using spinach, stir it in here along with additional sea salt and pepper if desired.
8. Top with grated cheese and enjoy.

Salads

Tahini Kale Salad
Sweet Curry Kale Pasta Salad
Classic Chicken Salad
Protein Power Salad Recipe
with Hemp Seeds & Sauerkraut
Sports Super Salad

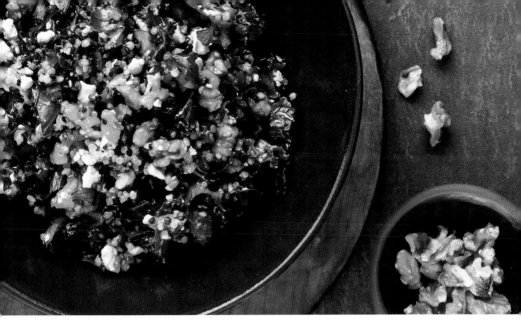

Tahini Kale Salad

COURSE Salad	**CUISINE** Mediterranean	**4 SERVINGS**	**COOK TIME** 4 minutes

Kale is a top superfood, filled with potassium, calcium, and Vitamin K. Some say it's bitter and difficult to eat, but add some garlic, almond butter, and apple cider vinegar with this Tahini Kale Salad recipe and you have a nutrient powerhouse salad that is easy to digest.

INGREDIENTS

- 2 bunches kale, stems removed and chopped
- 2-3 cloves garlic, minced or pressed
- 3-4 tbsp almond butter
- 2 tbsp olive oil, extra virgin
- 1 tbsp apple cider vinegar
- 1 tsp liquid aminos *(or tamari)*
- 1 lemon for juicing

OPTIONAL ADD-INS:

- nutritional yeast
- chickpeas
- raw cashews
- almonds sliced
- sesame seeds
- red onions, chopped
- hemp seeds

INSTRUCTIONS

1. Juice lemon
2. Mix ingredients together and enjoy!

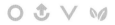

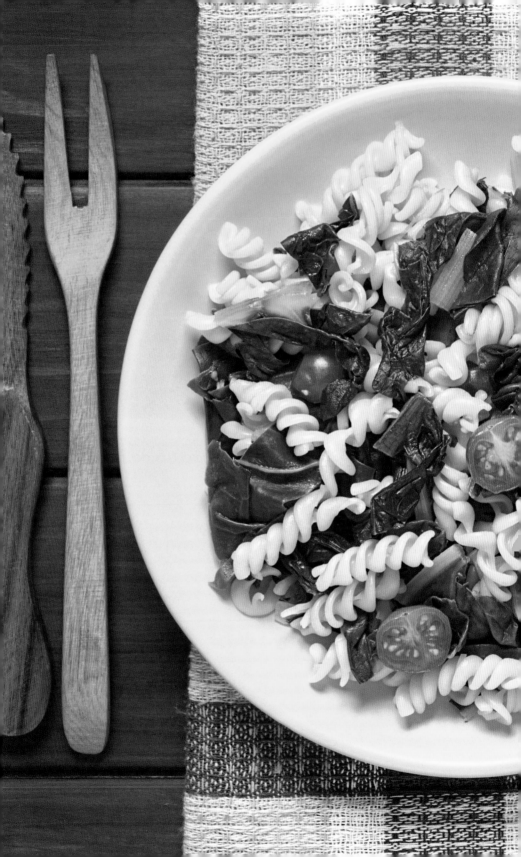

Sweet Curry Kale Pasta Salad

 COURSE
Salad

 CUISINE
American

 10 SERVINGS

 COOK TIME
2 hours

You will not believe that this salad is Core Plan! The pasta is made from 100% organic red lentils and nothing else. The flavored vinegars and oils mentioned below come locally and can typically be found at a market or health food store.

INGREDIENTS

SALAD:
- 12 oz. kale cleaned, ribbed, cut
- ¼ cup lemon or lime juice, freshly squeezed
- ¼ cup garlic infused olive oil (or olive oil)
- ¼- ½ tsp sea salt to taste
- fresh ground black pepper to taste
- 1 tsp curry powder
- ⅛- ¼ tsp stevia to taste
- 2 tbsp sesame seeds
- ¼ cup slivered almonds or other raw nuts

PASTA SALAD:
- 4 cup dry red lentil pasta
- ½ tsp sea salt
- 30 oz black beans organic, drained and rinsed
- ⅓ cup white balsamic vinegar (or other balsamic vinegar)
- ⅓ cup garlic infused olive oil or olive oil
- 2 tbsp additional garlic infused olive oil
- ¼ tsp sea salt
- fresh ground black pepper
- ½ small head of green or red cabbage

INSTRUCTIONS

1. Put kale in a large bowl and drizzle the lemon or lime juice over it. Set aside.
2. Come back periodically over the next 20 minutes to 2 hours to toss the kale. Alternately, you may also refrigerate the kale/juice mixture for up to a day and come back to toss periodically.
3. If you add other ingredients in as little as 20 minutes, it will still be very yummy, but the flavors will continue to improve over time.
4. When ready to add other salad ingredients, add them in the order listed and sprinkle each item over all the kale, stirring after addition of oil, and then again after the last ingredient.
5. Taste-test and adjust seasonings to your liking.
6. The kale will be ready by the time you have everything else put together.
7. Put the drained, rinsed beans into a medium bowl, sprinkle with the salt and pepper, mix.
8. Next add the ⅓ cup of vinegar and ⅓ cup of garlic olive oil and toss. Periodically toss this mixture also while assembling the remaining ingredients.
9. Next cook the pasta according to package directions, adding ½ teaspoon sea salt to the water. Do not overcook!
10. Drain and rinse, and return to the original cooking pot and let soak in cold filtered water (may add a few filtered ice cubes as well) until the pasta cools.
11. While the pasta cools, clean and slice the cabbage very thin using a knife, food processor slicing tool, or mandolin.
12. Drain the cooled pasta, toss with the additional 2 tablespoons of garlic olive oil, and add to the kale salad.
13. Next put the sliced cabbage on top of the pasta, followed by the marinated black bean mixture.
14. Toss, taste-test, adjust seasonings if necessary, and enjoy!

NOTE: *You can have fun with other variations of this salad adding other seed or nuts, or changing the flavor of the vinegar and oils.*

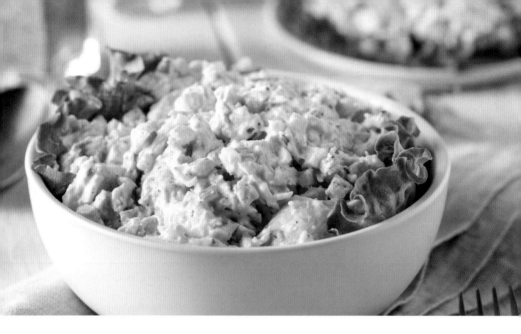

Classic Chicken Salad

 COURSE
Lunch

 CUISINE
American

 4 SERVINGS

 COOK TIME
30 minutes

Chicken salad is a popular lunch option, but standard recipes usually aren't very healthy. Try out our healthy spin on this hearty favorite—with only a few ingredients, it's packed with flavor. Top chicken salad on a sandwich, or enjoy it on its own.

INGREDIENTS

- 2 organic chicken breasts, cooked and chopped or shredded
- 1 cup organic plain Greek yogurt
- juice of ½ lemon
- ½ cup chopped nuts
- 2 stalks organic celery, chopped
- ½ onion, chopped
- 4 hearts of palm or artichokes, chopped

Optional: curry seasoning

Topping: chopped nuts/seeds of any assortment or gomashio

INSTRUCTIONS

1. Mix everything together and fill into an 8x8 baking dish.
2. Top with chopped nuts/seeds and bake at 350 degrees for 20 minutes, or until hot throughout.

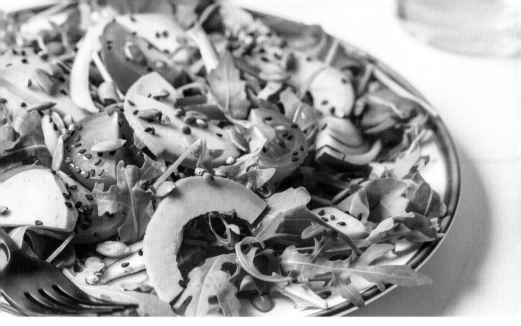

Protein Power Salad Recipe with Hemp Seeds & Sauerkraut

 COURSE
Salad

 CUISINE
American

 1 SERVING

 COOK TIME
5 minutes

Put a little power into your meal with this delicious salad. This easy plant-based protein salad is crunchy and tangy—the sauerkraut packs a flavorful punch! Although our salad recipe is vegan, you can top it with grilled wild fish or organic chicken. Customize this healthy salad with your favorite toppings—we recommend red onion, black olives, kelp granules, or sunflower sprouts!

INGREDIENTS

- 4 overflowing cups greens of your choice (like spinach or kale)
- 2 tbsp hemp seeds
- ½– 1 cup raw unpasteurized sauerkraut (look for the kind made and packed with water, not vinegar)
- 1 tbsp turmeric
- 1 handful raw nuts (use your favorite type)
- ½ avocado, sliced
- olive oil to taste
- apple cider vinegar to taste

Optional add-ins:
- ¼ red onion, chopped
- ⅓ cup black olives
- 2 tbsp kelp granules
- 1½ tsp sea salt (to taste)
- ¼ cup sunflower sprouts

INSTRUCTIONS

1. Mix all ingredients together and enjoy!

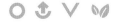

95

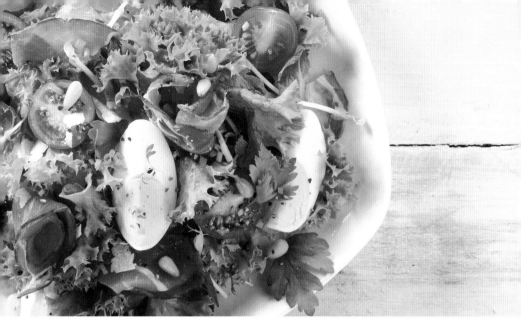

Sports Super Salad

 COURSE
Salad

 CUISINE
American

 1 SERVING

COOK TIME
5 minutes

Try this delicious take on a sports salad, with grass-fed beef and plenty of yummy greens.

INGREDIENTS

Salad Base:
- 1 head romaine lettuce or
- bowlful of baby mixed greens or baby spinach

Toppings:
- ½ chopped cucumber
- ½ cup chopped tomatoes
- 1 chopped avocado
- 1 grilled bison or grass-fed beef burger
- 2 hard boiled eggs, sliced

Dressing:
- hot pepper sauce (check label for no sugar)
- olive oil & balsamic vinegar
- homemade ranch dressing

INSTRUCTIONS

1. Mix all ingredients except burger in a large bowl or plate and top with a hot burger.
2. Drizzle with dressing.

Entrées

Wild Caught Cod Provencal
Salmon Almondine
Asian Salmon Skewers
Chicken Asparagus Marsala
Loaded Cauliflower Chicken Bake
Chicken Wings
Quick Chicken Spiedini and Green Beans
Tortilla Chip Chicken Casserole
One Pan Balsamic Chicken And Veggies
Grass-fed Steaks with Creamy Peppercorn Sauce
Tex-Mex Casserole with Corn-less Bread Topping
Apple Turkey Sausage Stuffed Acorn Squash
Cabbage Steaks
Basic Chili
Meatloaf
Spaghetti (Squash) with Meat Sauce
Shepherd's Pie
Roasted Vegetable Lasagna

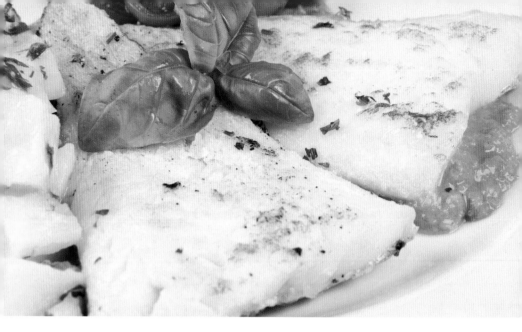

Wild Caught Cod Provencal

 COURSE
Main Course

 CUISINE
Mediterranean

 4 SERVINGS

 COOK TIME
15 minutes

This is a very simple yet elegant way to serve fish. Herbs de Provence is a spice mixture originating in France that contains a combination of savory, marjoram, rosemary, thyme, oregano and lavender. You can find it at most grocery stores and specialty stores. It gives the fish a very unique and exotic flavor.

INGREDIENTS

- 4 Pacific cod filets, large, wild-caught
- 2 tbsp dijon mustard
- 1 tsp dried herbs de Provence
- 1 tsp fresh garlic, chopped
- 2 tbsp avocado oil or melted coconut oil
- 2 handfuls organic cherry tomatoes *(optional)*
- sea salt
- black pepper

INSTRUCTIONS

1. Preheat oven to 450 degrees.
2. Combine mustard, herbs de Provence, garlic, and oil.
3. Brush over fish and let marinate for 30 minutes in the refrigerator.
4. Place fish in a glass baking dish.
5. Scatter cherry tomatoes around the fish, if desired and sprinkle everything with more herbs de Provence, sea salt, and pepper.
6. Cook for 12-15 minutes or until cod flakes with a fork.

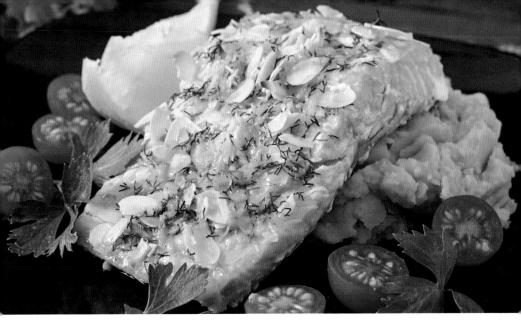

Salmon Almondine

COURSE Main Course	**CUISINE** American	**2 SERVINGS**	**COOK TIME** 35 minutes

This is a delicious and beautiful way to serve salmon. Because it is sliced thin, it cooks in just a few minutes. The simple ingredients come together wonderfully for a very flavorful dish. The sour burst from the capers and the crunch from the almonds make it truly unique.

INGREDIENTS

- 3 tbsp butter, grass-fed
- 1 tsp avocado oil
- ¼ cup almonds, sliced
- 14 oz wild-caught salmon (fillet cut into 1/4-inch-wide slices)
- ½ juice lemon
- 1 tbsp capers, drained

INSTRUCTIONS

1. Melt 1 tablespoon butter and 1 teaspoon avocado oil in a nontoxic skillet over medium heat.
2. Lightly brown the almonds; set aside.
3. Season salmon with salt and pepper.
4. Cook 1 at a time. Saute on both sides until done.
5. Saute the other salmon fillet.
6. Add another 2 tablespoons of grass-fed butter, lemon juice, and capers.
7. Put the mixture on a plate and drizzle with any remaining sauce in the pan.
8. Sprinkle with the almonds and serve immediately.

NOTE: *Keep whole nutmeg in your freezer and use a microplane to grate it fresh for recipes. The taste is amazing and the nutmeg will last virtually forever in the freezer.*

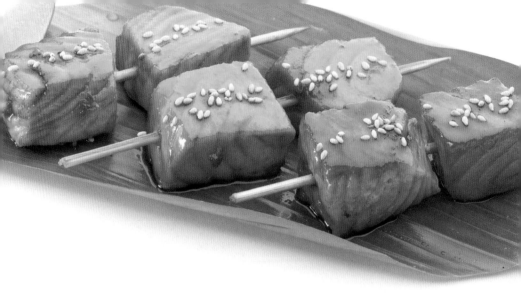

Asian Salmon Skewers

 COURSE
Main Course

 CUISINE
Asian

 3 SERVINGS

 COOK TIME
1 hour 10 minutes

These Asian Salmon Skewers are quick and easy to make and beautifully presented. Kids and adults will love this dish; it is great served with sautéed bok choy with ginger and brown rice or cauliflower rice.

INGREDIENTS

- 1 clove garlic, minced
- 1 inch piece ginger, microplaned
- 1 lime (zested and juiced)
- 3 tbsp coconut aminos or liquid aminos
- 1 tsp olive oil, extra virgin
- 2 fillets wild caught salmon cut into 1" chunks
- 1 tbsp sesame seeds *(optional, toasted)*
- 1 package bamboo skewers

INSTRUCTIONS

1. Soak mini bamboo skewers in water for 30+ minutes to prevent burning.
2. Prepare the marinade by combining the garlic, ginger, ½ of the zest, ½ of the juice (you can save the remaining for rice, veggies, or other use), aminos, honey, and olive oil.
3. Add the salmon chunks and carefully coat with marinade. Marinate at least 15 minutes.
4. Skewer the salmon onto bamboo skewers and grill on an outdoor or indoor grill pan for 8-10 minutes, turning frequently and basting with remaining marinade.
5. Toast sesame seeds in a dry pan, if desired and sprinkle over salmon and serve.

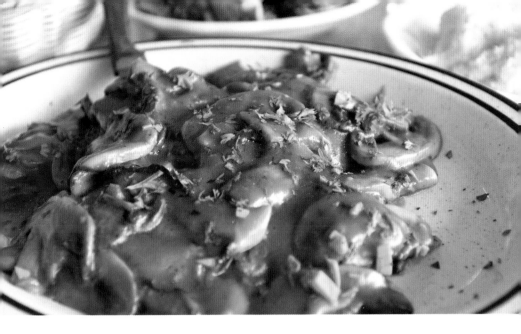

Chicken Asparagus Marsala

 COURSE
Main Course

 CUISINE
American, Italian

 6 SERVINGS

 COOK TIME
17 minutes

Asparagus always give a dish an elegant flair. Here, it also adds beautiful color.

INGREDIENTS

- 4 free range chicken-breast, halves, boned and skinned
- 10 oz asparagus spears, cut
- 2 tbsp butter
- 1 tbsp coconut (or grapeseed oil)
- ½ lbs mushrooms
- ¼ cup marsala wine
- ½ tsp salt
- ¼ cup water
- ⅛ tsp pepper
- 1 tbsp parsley, chopped diagonally into pieces

INSTRUCTIONS

1. Pound the chicken pieces to ¼-inch thickness.
2. Melt the butter in a frying pan over medium-high temperature.
3. Add chicken and cook, turning, for about 5 minutes or until the chicken is brown.
4. Remove chicken and set aside.
5. To the drippings remaining in the frying pan, add the asparagus and mushrooms and cook, stirring, for about 3 minutes.
6. Return the chicken to the pan, add the marsala wine, water, salt, and pepper.
7. Bring the mixture to a boil for 2 minutes to reduce the liquid.
8. Reduce heat, cover and simmer for about 3 minutes or until the chicken and vegetables are tender.
9. Arrange the chicken on a serving platter.
10. Spoon the vegetable sauce over the chicken.
11. Sprinkle with chopped parsley and serve.

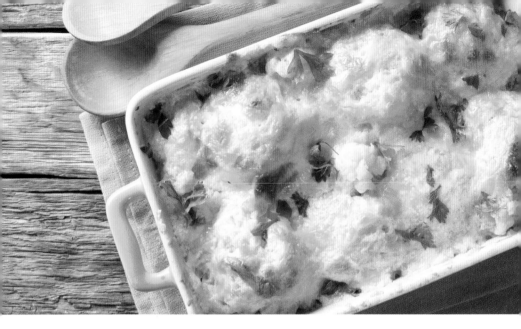

Loaded Cauliflower Chicken Bake

 COURSE
Main Course

 CUISINE
American

 8 SERVINGS

 COOK TIME
50 minutes

This recipe was inspired to give people a healthy dish to enjoy at their Super Bowl parties. It was so simple to make and was a hit with the family. It somewhat resembles a loaded baked potato but uses cauliflower instead of potatoes. It would be great to bring to any potluck or family event. If you are trying to avoid dairy, you can add nutritional yeast to the top instead of cheese.

INGREDIENTS

- 1-1 ½ lb organic chicken thighs or breasts cut into large chunks
- 1 head organic cauliflower, cut into florets
- 1 tbsp high quality paprika
- 1 tbsp garlic powder
- ¼ cup olive oil
- 2 tbsp hot pepper sauce (check ingredients)
- ¼ tsp sea salt
- 1 lb turkey bacon, cooked and chopped
- 1-2 cup organic grass-fed cheddar cheese
- 1-2 green onions, chopped

INSTRUCTIONS

1. Mix the olive oil, paprika, garlic powder and hot pepper sauce together in a large bowl.
2. Add cauliflower and chicken and mix until everything is covered with the spice mixture.
3. Put into a large glass baking dish and cook at 425 degrees for about 40 minutes.
4. Top with grated cheese and bacon and place back in the oven until the cheese is melted.
5. Sprinkle with green onions and serve.

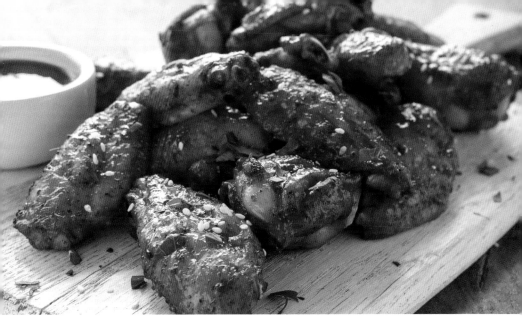

Chicken Wings

 COURSE
Main Course

 CUISINE
American

 4 SERVINGS

 COOK TIME
35 minutes

No deep fryer for these delicious chicken wings. No hydrogenated oils, and no resulting stomach aches. Plus, enjoy the easy preparation with just a saucepan and one bowl! Easy, healthy family dinner or for one.

INGREDIENTS

- ¼ cup unsalted butter, grass-fed, organic
- 1 tsp granulated stevia
- ¼ cup red wine (optional)
- ¼ cup liquid aminos (or organic tamari)
- 2 tbsp fresh lemon juice
- 1 tsp dijon mustard
- ⅛ cup hot sauce (adjust to your taste)
- 2 lbs organic chicken wings
- 1 tsp sea salt
- ⅛ tsp black pepper
- 1 tsp garlic powder

INSTRUCTIONS

1. Preheat oven to 350° F.
2. Melt butter in a small-medium sauce pan over medium heat.
3. Add the stevia, wine, tamara, lemon juice, dijon, hot sauce, salt, pepper and garlic powder to the sauce pan and mix. Simmer until wine cooks down.
4. In a large bowl, pour the sauce over the wings.
5. Arrange chicken wings on a large baking sheet lined with parchment paper.
6. Bake wings at 350° F for 35-40 minutes, or until chicken is cooked through.
7. NOTE: For even more tender wings with a further reduced sauce, reduce heat to 250° F degrees and continue cooking for 3-4 hours, flipping every 30 minutes.

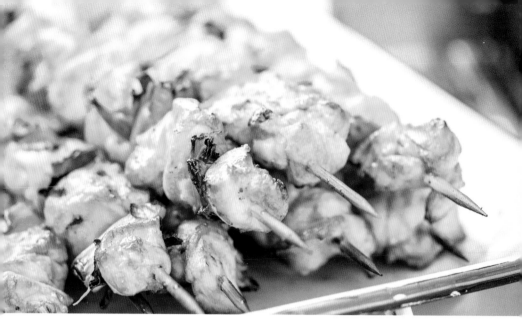

Quick Chicken Spiedini and Green Beans

 COURSE
Main Course

 CUISINE
Italian, Mediterranean

 3 SERVINGS

 PREP TIME **COOK TIME**
30 minutes 8 minutes

This recipe was born out of an unplanned dinner. It is the result of the art of cooking-taking random ingredients and making them into delicious meals. This recipe is a total home run with the family!

INGREDIENTS

- 2 lbs boneless organic chicken breasts, cut into 1" chunks
- 2 juice of lemons
- 1 zest of lemon
- ½ tsp dried rosemary or 1 tsp fresh rosemary
- ¼ cup olive oil
- sea salt to taste
- fresh ground black pepper to taste
- crushed red pepper *(optional)*

INSTRUCTIONS

1. Mix all ingredients and let marinate at least 30 minutes to overnight.
2. Place 5-6 chunks of chicken on pre-soaked wooden skewers (soak them so that they don't catch on fire).
3. Cook on an outdoor grill or indoor cast iron grill pan until no longer pink inside.
4. Garnish with additional lemon zest if desired.

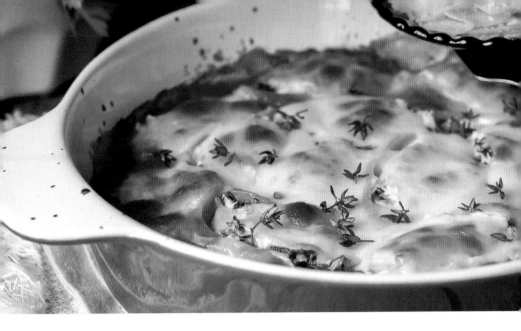

Tortilla Chip Chicken Casserole

 COURSE
Main Course

 CUISINE
Tex-Mex

 8 SERVINGS

 COOK TIME
30 minutes

This is a quick and simple dish that is hearty and satisfying. By cooking the whole chicken, you get more flavor and nutrients and can save the bones to make homemade chicken broth.

INGREDIENTS

- 2 cup chopped, free range chicken
- ¼ large onion, chopped
- 2 garlic cloves, minced
- 1½ tbsp chipotle peppers in adobo sauce, minced
- 1¾ cup free-range chicken broth or cream of chicken soup, check ingredients
- 1 cup water
- 1 tomato cored, seeded and chopped
- 1 tsp sea salt
- 1½ cup grass-fed cheddar cheese, shredded
- 1 bag grain-free tortilla chips
- ¼ cup black olives, sliced
- 2 tbsp fresh cilantro, chopped (optional)
- guacamole if desired
- organic sour cream as garnish

INSTRUCTIONS

1. Preheat oven to 350° F. degrees.
2. Cook the chicken (can be done in an InstantPot) and set aside.
3. Put onion, garlic, chipotle peppers, broth or soup, tomato, and salt in a blender and mix into a smooth sauce.
4. Put a layer of chips in a casserole dish.
5. Top with half of the chicken and half of the sauce.
6. Sprinkle a light layer of cheese then repeat with another layer of chips, sauce and cheese and sprinkle with sliced black olives, if desired.
7. Bake for 30 minutes or until bubbly. Top with cilantro and serve hot.

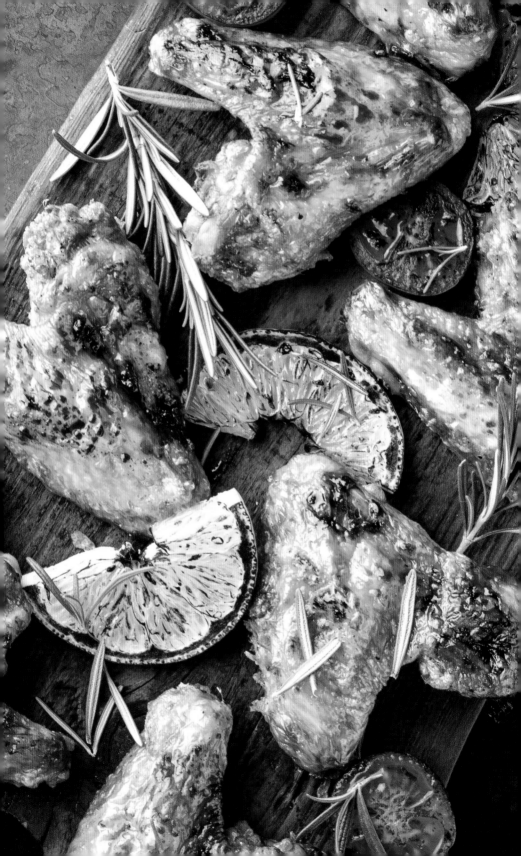

One Pan Balsamic Chicken And Veggies

 COURSE
Main Course

 CUISINE
American,
Mediterranean

 6 SERVINGS

COOK TIME
30 minutes

This is a great go-to recipe that is wonderful for busy nights or to use up any extra vegetables you have on hand. It also makes for great leftovers. As an added bonus, there is only one pan to wash!

INGREDIENTS

- 2 lbs. organic chicken breasts
- 1 head broccoli, cut into florets
- 1 head cauliflower, cut into florets
- 3 carrots, cut into sticks *(core plan only)*
- 2 cup mushrooms
- 1 red onion, chopped into chunks
- ⅓ cup grape or cherry tomatoes organic
- ½ cup balsamic vinegar, plus more for drizzling

- ¼ cup avocado or melted coconut oil, plus more for drizzling
- 4 cloves garlic, minced
- 3-4 tbsp fresh basil, chopped
- 1 tsp fresh thyme or ½ teaspoon dried thyme
- ½ tsp sea salt
- ¼ tsp black pepper

INSTRUCTIONS

1. Preheat oven to 400° F. Line two baking sheets with parchment paper.
2. Combine balsamic vinegar, oil, garlic, basil, thyme, salt and pepper. Whisk.
3. Place chicken in a bowl and pour balsamic mixture over the chicken and mix well.
4. Put into the refrigerator while preparing the vegetables, you can do this earlier for even more flavor.
5. Chop all of the vegetables and place on the sheet pan (leave out the cherry tomatoes for now as they cook faster).
6. Drizzle with a little more oil and balsamic vinegar and sprinkle with salt/pepper. Mix well.
7. Remove the chicken from the marinade and move vegetables around so that you can fit the chicken in. Place chicken on the pan.
8. Bake for 10 minutes, remove from oven and add tomatoes, cook for 10-20 more minutes, depending on the thickness of the chicken.

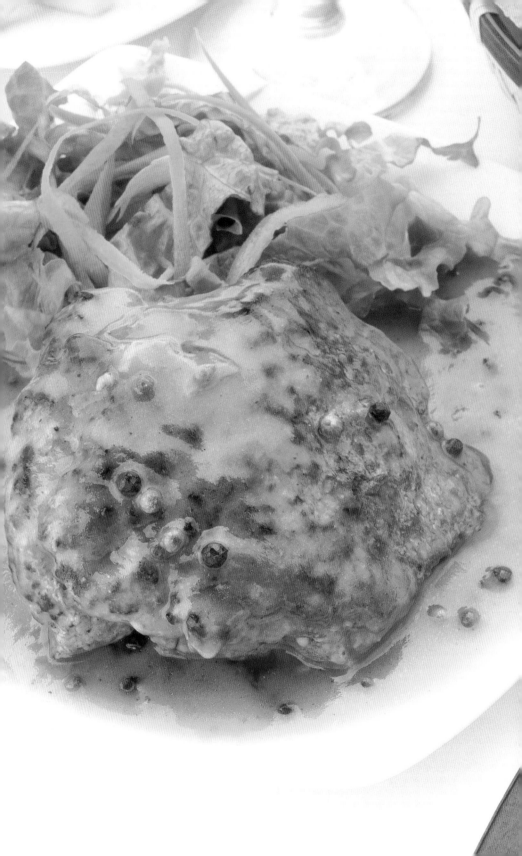

Grass-Fed Steaks with Creamy Peppercorn Sauce

 COURSE
Main Course

 CUISINE
American

 4 SERVINGS

COOK TIME
15 minutes

Grass fed beef steaks are a culinary delight. They are far superior to conventional beef—in nutrition, in taste, and for the environment. This is a great alternative to grilling steaks outside and the sauce is outstanding. It makes for a beautiful presentation so it would be perfect for guests.

INGREDIENTS

- 1-2 tbsp freshly ground whole peppercorns with a course grind
- 4 grass-fed steaks fillet or NY strip
- 1 tsp sea salt
- 2 tbsp grass-fed butter
- 1 tbsp avocado oil (or coconut oil)

- 1 large shallot, finely chopped
- ⅓ cup grass-fed beef broth, homemade or store bought
- 1 cup heavy cream, organic

INSTRUCTIONS

1. Sprinkle both sides of the steak with salt and crushed peppercorns.
2. Press the peppercorns into the steaks.
3. In a large, heavy non-toxic skillet (cast iron works best), melt the butter and avocado oil (do not let the butter smoke).
4. Cook steaks until desired doneness. A 6 oz steak will typically take about 3 minutes on each side. When done, transfer to a dish and cover.
5. Add a little more oil if necessary and cook shallot until soft (a minute or two).
6. Add the remaining butter and melt. Pour in the broth and let cook for another minute.
7. Add heavy cream and stir frequently until reduced to a thick sauce (6-7 minutes).
8. Add a pinch or two of sea salt and taste for appropriate seasoning. Return steaks (and any juices that escaped) back into the skillet and cover well with sauce. Serve with any remaining sauce.

NOTE: *Grass-fed beef is best cooked rare—medium rare.*
Great served with mashed cauliflower and oven roasted broccoli.

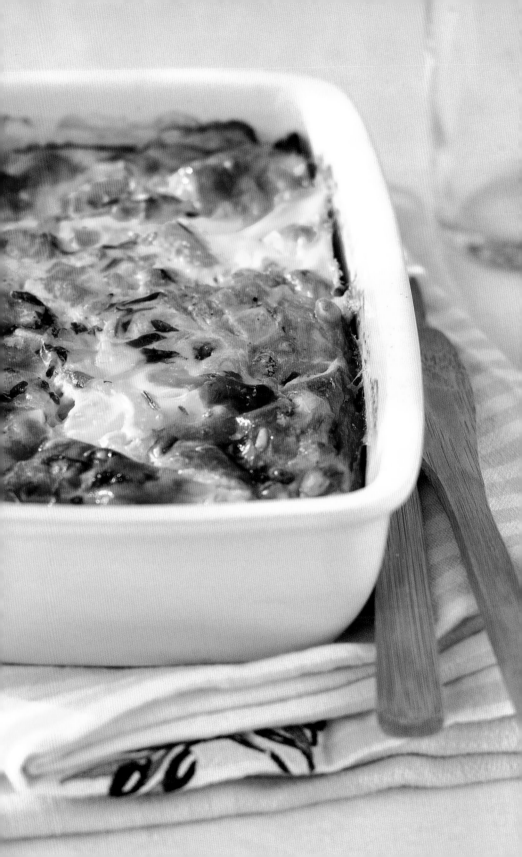

Tex-Mex Casserole with Corn-less Bread Topping

 COURSE
Main Course

 CUISINE
Tex-Mex

 8 SERVINGS

 COOK TIME
50 minutes

A casserole is a great easy-to-make, dish to bring to a potluck or social event. The Tex-Mex Casserole with Corn-less Bread Topping is versatile too, since you can leave out or add any veggies you have on hand or make it a completely vegetarian dish by leaving out the beef. This recipe is by Dr. Rosie Main.

INGREDIENTS

CASSEROLE:
- 1 tbsp chili powder
- 1½ tsp ground cumin
- 1 tsp sweet paprika, smoked
- ½ tsp cayenne pepper more to taste, if desired
- 1¼ tsp sea salt
- ½ tsp ground coriander (*optional*)
- 2 lb grass-fed ground beef
- ½ red onion, diced
- ½ organic zucchini, diced
- 2 cloves garlic, minced
- 1 organic bell pepper, diced
- 1 jalapeño, seeded and diced (optional)
- Fine-grain sea salt and freshly ground black pepper to taste

- 1 large tomato, seeded and diced or 1 (14 oz) can diced tomatoes, with their juices
- 1 cup tomato sauce or tomato puree
- 2 cup kale leaves (or baby spinach), chopped
- 1 can sliced black olives (save a handful for topping)
- 15 oz can black beans, drained and rinsed
- 1 tsp arrowroot powder
- ¼ cup filtered water

OPTIONAL TOPPINGS:
- Sliced green onions
- Salsa
- Avocado

CORN-LESS BREAD TOPPING:
- 1 cup almond flour
- ¾ tsp baking powder
- ½ tsp sea salt
- 2 large eggs, organic, cage free
- 2 tbsp butter, softened
- ¼ cup grass-fed plain yogurt or full fat coconut milk

OPTIONAL:
- 2 green onions ,chopped
- 1 jalapeño, seeded and chopped

INSTRUCTIONS

CORN-LESS BREAD TOPPING:
1. Preheat the oven to 350° F.
2. Brown the grass-fed ground beef with the onions, zucchini, garlic, and bell pepper.
3. Meanwhile, mix the chili powder, cumin, paprika, salt, and coriander in a small bowl.
4. When beef is browned and vegetables are softened, drain any excess grease from the pan.
5. Add in jalapeño, salt/pepper, tomato and tomato sauce, kale, black olives, and black beans.
6. Mix the arrowroot powder with filtered water and mix well then add to the pan and mix all ingredients.
7. Transfer the mixture to a large cast iron pan or glass baking dish.
8. Top with Corn-less Cornbread mixture and bake for 30 minutes at 350° F or until cornbread is browned around the edges.

CORN-LESS BREAD:
1. Preheat the oven to 350° F.
2. In a bowl, mix yogurt or coconut milk, softened butter and eggs.
3. Add the almond flour, baking powder and salt and mix again.
4. Mix in the chopped green onions.
5. Pour into a greased 8 inch glass baking dish and bake for 20 minutes or until the edges and top are slightly browned.

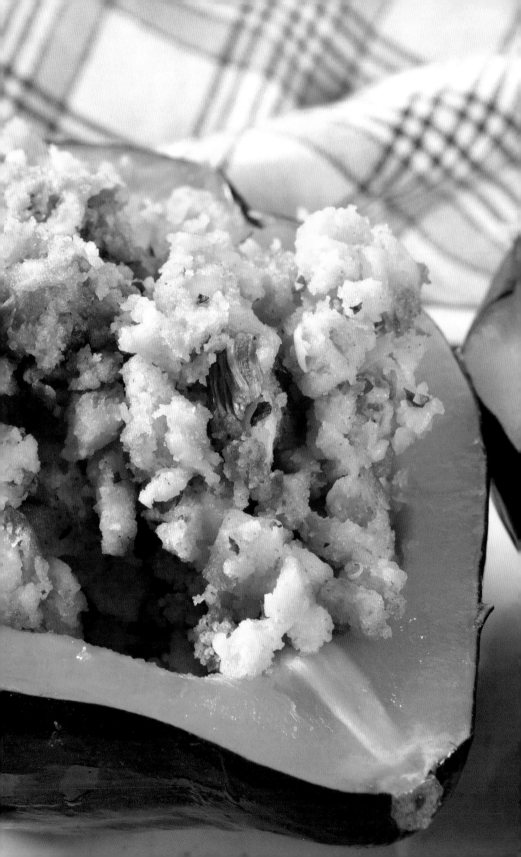

Apple Turkey Sausage Stuffed Acorn Squash

 COURSE
Main Course

 CUISINE
American

6 SERVINGS

COOK TIME
53 minutes

This is a great fall recipe! It comes together really quickly and makes for a beautiful presentation (don't you love how fruits and vegetables look so amazing?). This is an Advanced Plan recipe that makes you fall more in love with your commitment to eating well. This should end up in your recipe rotation.

INGREDIENTS

- 3 acorn squash
- avocado or coconut oil, as needed
- dried Italian seasoning to taste
- sea salt to taste
- cayenne pepper *(optional)*
- 1 lb mild Italian turkey or chicken sausage
- 1 small onion, finely diced
- 2 ribs celery, finely diced
- 1 large granny smith apple, diced
- 1 cup shredded parmesan cheese *(optional: leave out for a dairy-free alternative)*

INSTRUCTIONS

1. Preheat the oven to 425°F.
2. Cut the stem end and the bottom ends (as little as possible) of each of the squash.
3. Cut them in half (they should easily stand up). Scoop out the seeds with a spoon and discard. Put on a parchment lined baking dish.
4. Drizzle with avocado or coconut oil and sprinkle with Italian seasoning, sea salt, and cayenne pepper if desired.
5. Bake for about 40 minutes or until soft to the fork (don't overcook as it will lose its shape).
6. Cut casings off of sausage and saute in a pan with onions and celery.
7. Break up the sausage into small bits. When browned, add the apple and saute for 2-3 more minutes. Stir in ¾ cup parmesan cheese.
8. Put mixture in the acorn squash and sprinkle with additional parmesan back in the oven for about 10 minutes.
9. Serve hot.

NOTE: *Squash should be eaten in moderation on the Advanced Plan and it is fine on the Core Plan.*

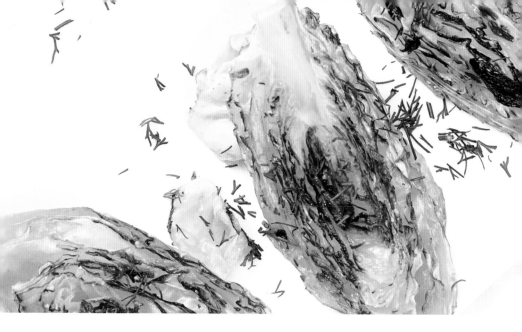

Cabbage Steaks

 COURSE
Main Course

 CUISINE
American

5 SERVINGS

COOK TIME
15 minutes

Cabbage steaks are a yummy alternative for when you want a browned steak-like dish, but are looking for a healthier option. These cabbage steaks are both delicious and good for you, too!

INGREDIENTS

- ⅓ cup avocado oil or coconut oil
- 1 head green cabbage
- 1 tsp sea salt
- 1 tsp garlic powder
- 1 tsp paprika
- ½ tsp onion powder
- ¼ tsp ground pepper

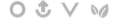

INSTRUCTIONS

1. Preheat the oven to 425°F degrees.
2. Slice cabbage into circles, trying to keep the core attached to the leaves (this keeps the steaks from falling apart). Some of the end pieces may be loose but cook them anyway.
3. Rub a large baking sheet with oil while you preheat the oven.
4. Slice cabbage and place on baking sheet.
5. Brush each cabbage slice with oil and sprinkle with spices.
6. Roast for until edges are caramelized and becoming crispy. Depending on how thick your slices are will determine cooking time. Check after 15 minutes and adjust time from there.

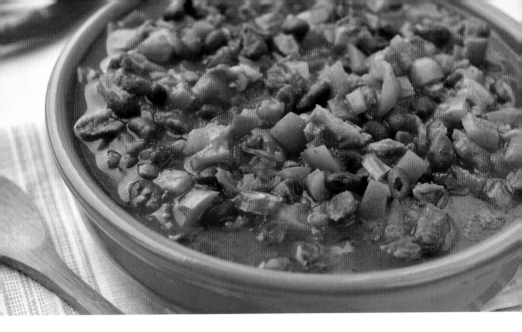

Basic Chili

 COURSE
Lunch, Main Course

 CUISINE
American

 5 SERVINGS

 COOK TIME
1 hour 10 minutes

Everyone should have this chili recipe in their collection because it's the perfect easy chili! It is healthy, easy to make, and travels well. You can also use this recipe to make a fun taco salad. Just pour over mixed greens with your favorite toppings.

INGREDIENTS

- 1 tbsp coconut oil
- ½ cup onion, chopped or grated
- ½ cup celery, chopped
- 2 cloves garlic, minced
- 1 cup green pepper, chopped
- 1 can kidney beans or black beans
- 2 tsp oregano
- 2 tsp chili powder
- 2 tsp ground cumin
- 1 tsp sea salt
- 8 oz canned organic crushed tomatoes
- 1-1½ lb ground bison, grass-fed beef, or ground turkey
- 1 small jalapeno seeded and chopped finely *(optional)*

INSTRUCTIONS

1. In a large, deep skillet melt oil and sauté onions, celery, garlic, peppers and jalapeno, until onion is translucent (3-4 minutes).
2. Add ground meat, oregano, chili powder, and cumin, continue cooking, stirring frequently (5-6 minutes).
3. Then, pour salt and tomatoes into pot.
4. Cover and reduce heat, then simmer for a minimum of 1 hour for best flavor.

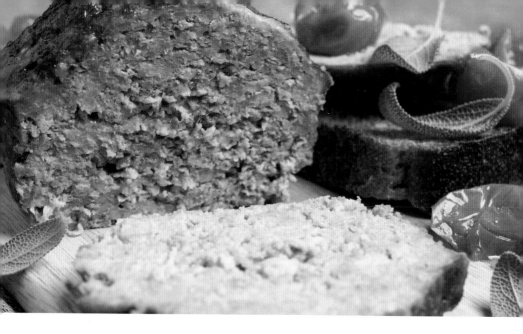

Meatloaf

 COURSE
Main Course

 CUISINE
American

 6-8 SERVINGS

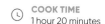 **COOK TIME**
1 hour 20 minutes

Here is another traditional favorite that everyone will love.

INGREDIENTS

- 1 lb grass-fed ground beef
- 1 small yellow onion chopped
- 1 clove garlic, minced
- ½ cup flat leaf parsley, finely chopped
- 1 large cage free egg, lightly beaten
- 1 cup sprouted grain bread, lightly toasted and processed into crumbs
- ⅔ cup organic tomato paste or ketchup *(no sugar)*
- 1 tsp sea salt
- ½ tsp pepper

INSTRUCTIONS

1. Preheat oven to 375°F.
2. In a medium bowl, combine chopped onion, garlic, parsley, egg, and ⅓ cup ketchup.
3. Add breadcrumbs and beef. Season with salt and pepper. Mix until well combined.
4. Place mixture in a 6 cup capacity loaf pan (8 x 4 in) or simply shape into a loaf in a glass baking dish. Pat gently to make a rounded top. Do not pack.
5. Bake meatloaf 50 minutes. Remove from oven; brush with remaining ⅓ cup tomato paste or ketchup.
6. Return to the oven; bake until an instant-read thermometer inserted into the center of the loaf reads 160°F, approximately 10 – 20 minutes.
7. Cool meatloaf for 10 minutes in the pan before slicing.

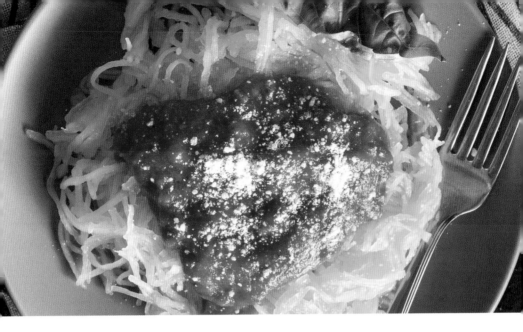

Spaghetti (Squash) with Meat Sauce

 COURSE
Main Course

 CUISINE
Italian

 4 SERVINGS

 COOK TIME
1 hour

This delicious spaghetti dish has no pasta. Create the perfect Italian meal with spaghetti squash and up your protein with meat sauce. Make for dinner or for lunch.

INGREDIENTS

- 2 large spaghetti squash
- 2 jars pasta sauce *(16 oz jars, check ingredients for no sugar or MSG)*
- 1 lb grass-fed ground beef *(with seasoning, sea salt, pepper, garlic)*

INSTRUCTIONS

1. Cut the spaghetti squash in half and scoop out seeds.
2. Put about ½ inch of water in a baking dish and place squash, cut sides down, in the dish.
3. Bake for about 45-60 minutes depending on the size of the squash or until soft. (Do not overcook).
4. Flip the squash over and use a fork to loosen the "noodles".
5. Brown ground beef with seasoning, drain and add pasta sauce.

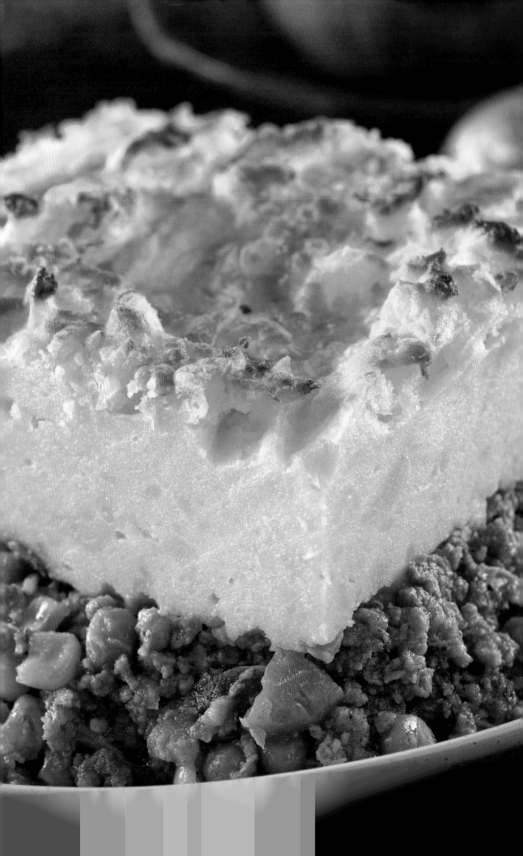

Shepherd's Pie

 COURSE
Main Course

 CUISINE
English

4 SERVINGS

COOK TIME
20 minutes

This version of shepherd's pie is made without the traditional starchy potatoes and uses mashed cauliflower instead. It also contains grass fed beef, making it an ultra-healthy alternative to traditional shepherd's pie. It tastes very close to the original. It also makes for a great presentation.

INGREDIENTS

Mashed Cauliflower:
- 1 head cauliflower
- ½ tsp minced garlic
- 2 tbsp organic butter
- ½ tsp salt
- ⅛ tsp freshly ground pepper
- 1 organic egg yolk

Pie Filling:
- 1 tbsp coconut oil or grapeseed oil
- 2 lbs grass-fed ground beef
- 1 tsp sea salt
- ½ tsp freshly ground pepper
- 1 carrot, peeled and chopped
- ½ large onion, chopped
- 2 tbsp organic butter
- 1 tsp xanthan gum *(thickener)*
- 1 cup organic vegetable broth
- 1 tsp wheat-free tamari
- ½ cup frozen peas *(optional)*

INSTRUCTIONS

1. Steam cauliflower until soft then transfer to a food processor or blender.
2. Puree the cauliflower with the garlic, butter, salt, pepper, and egg yolk.
3. While the cauliflower is steaming, preheat a large skillet over medium high heat.
4. Add oil to pan with beef. Season meat with salt and pepper and brown with carrot and onion until the meat is no longer pink.
5. In a separate saucepan cook butter and xanthan gum together combining well. Whisk in broth and tamari. Thicken gravy about 1 minute.
6. Add gravy to meat and vegetables and stir in the peas.
7. Preheat broiler to high.
8. Put meat mixture into a rectangular or round baking dish and spread cauliflower over the meat as evenly as possible being careful not to let meat show through.
9. Broil 6 to 8 inches from the heat until potatoes are evenly browned.

NOTE: *For Advanced Plan, leave out carrots and peas*

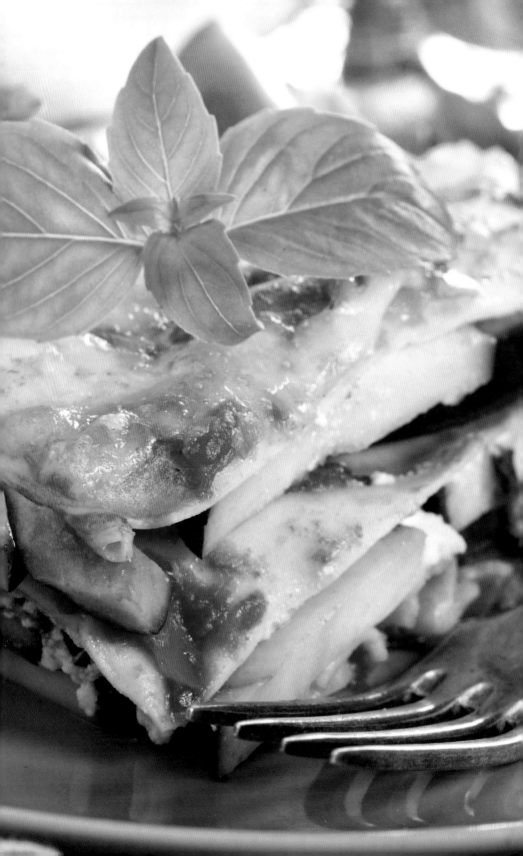

Roasted Vegetable Lasagna

 COURSE
Main Course

 CUISINE
Italian

 6 SERVINGS

 COOK TIME
1 hour 5 minutes

This meat-free, vegetarian lasagna uses eggplant, zucchini, and homemade, zero-sugar pasta sauce to create a hearty, healthy meal. With protein from egg and cheese, healthy fats, and garlic and pepper, this vegetarian lasagna recipe boosts your immune system and metabolism.

INGREDIENTS

- 1 large eggplant, sliced into ¼ inch rounds
- ½ lb mushrooms, sliced
- 3 small organic zucchini, sliced lengthwise into ¼ inch slices
- 2 organic red bell peppers
- 3 tbsp olive oil extra virgin
- 1 clove garlic, minced
- 15 oz organic ricotta cheese
- ½ tsp pepper, ground
- ¼ cup parmesan cheese, grated
- 1 organic egg
- 1 tsp sea salt
- 26 oz pasta sauce *(or homemade, check store jar ingredients – look for NO sugar)*
- 2 cup organic mozzarella cheese, grated
- 3 tbsp basil, minced

INSTRUCTIONS

1. Spread eggplant and mushrooms on a parchment lined baking sheet.
2. Place zucchini and red pepper on a second sheet.
3. Combine oil and garlic, then spread over both trays of vegetables.
4. Sprinkle both trays with salt and pepper.
5. Bake uncovered at 400° F for 15 minutes.
6. Turn vegetables over and cook until soft.
7. In a bowl, combine the ricotta cheese, parmesan cheese, and egg.
8. Spread about ½ of the pasta sauce in a 9 in x 13 in glass baking dish.
9. Layer with half the ricotta cheese mixture, half of the vegetables, a third of the pasta sauce, and ⅔ of the mozzarella cheese.
10. Sprinkle with basil if desired.
11. Repeat layers.
12. Top with remaining pasta sauce and cheese. Cover, then bake at 350° F for about 40 minutes.
13. Uncover, sprinkle with remaining cheese. Bake 5–10 minutes longer or until edges are bubbly and cheese is melted.
14. Let stand for 10 minutes before cutting.

Sides & Appetizers

Asian Turkey Lettuce Wrap
Easy Stuffed Mushrooms
Philly Cheesesteak Stuffed Green Peppers
Zesty Lemon Quinoa
Braised Fennel
Delicate Brussels Sprouts Sautée
Blasted Cauliflower
Green Beans with Crushed Walnuts
Chile-Zucchini Mash
Optimal Energy Bar
Healthy Hummus

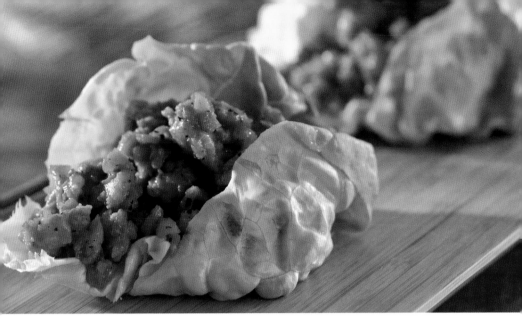

Asian Turkey Lettuce Wraps

 COURSE
Appetizer, Lunch

 CUISINE
Chinese

 3 SERVINGS

 COOK TIME
12 minutes

This is a very tasty lettuce wrap recipe, that rivals any Chinese takeout or even an elegant Chinese restaurant. It makes a nice presentation for an appetizer, as well.

INGREDIENTS

- ⅓ cups water
- 3 tbsp organic almond/ cashew butter
- 1 lb ground turkey
- 1 tbsp coconut oil
- 1 cup shiitake mushroom caps, chopped
- 1 tbsp rice vinegar
- 8 oz can of water chestnuts, drained and chopped
- 3 cloves garlic minced
- 2 tbsp ginger minced
- ⅓ cup tamari
- ½ cup green onions *(optional)*
- 1 head lettuce, separated into leaves

INSTRUCTIONS

1. Cook turkey in skillet with almond butter and coconut oil for about 5 minutes, stirring until turkey crumbles and is no longer pink.
2. Add mushrooms, rice vinegar, water chestnuts, garlic, ginger and tamari. Increase heat to medium-high, and cook, stirring constantly, for 4 minutes.
3. Add green onions if desired and cook, stirring constantly, for 1 minute.
4. Pull lettuce into leaves, if not done already.
5. Spoon mixture evenly onto lettuce leaves; roll up.
6. Serve with extra tamari sauce if desired.

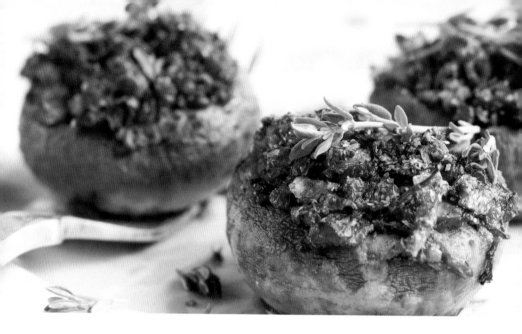

Easy Stuffed Mushrooms

 COURSE
Appetizer

 CUISINE
American

 5 SERVINGS

 COOK TIME
20 minutes

This stuffed mushroom recipe requires only three ingredients, takes a few minutes to make, and tastes delicious. Tasty and savory, there are sure to be no leftovers when you make these bacon and cheese stuffed mushrooms! They're perfect for entertaining—serve these delectable stuffed mushroom caps at your next party as an appetizer or quick snack. Core Plan approved.

INGREDIENTS

- 1 pint button or baby bella mushrooms (stems removed and cleaned with a damp towel)
- ½ brick organic cream cheese, softened (4 oz)
- 6 slices uncured turkey bacon, cooked and cut into small pieces

INSTRUCTIONS

1. Preheat oven to 350° F.
2. Mix the cream cheese with the chopped bacon and fill each mushroom cap. You will want a small mound on top.
3. Bake for 15–20 minutes on a parchment (or silicone baking mat) lined baking sheet. Serve warm or at room temperature.

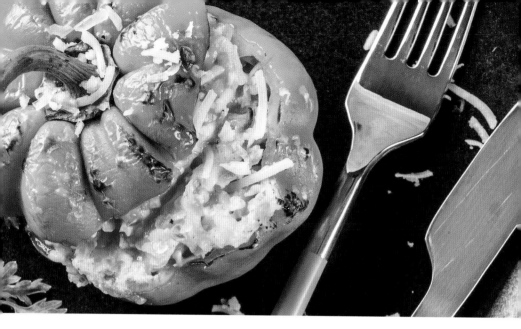

Philly Cheesesteak Stuffed Green Peppers

 COURSE
Main Course

 CUISINE
American

 4 SERVINGS

 COOK TIME
30 minutes

Craving a philly cheesesteak sandwich but don't want to load up on bread? This stuffed bell pepper recipe is the perfect alternative—a healthy version of a classic philly cheesesteak recipe without the bread or the mess! With grass-fed ground beef, mushrooms, onions, and cheese, these just might be the best-stuffed peppers you've ever had. Try this healthy gluten-free recipe tonight and let us know what you think.

INGREDIENTS

- 1 lb grass-fed ground beef
- 1 tsp sea salt
- ½ tsp black pepper
- 2 tsp liquid aminos or tamari
- 4–6 organic green bell peppers (tops cut off and ribs and seeds cleaned out)
- 4-6 organic green bell pepper, tops chopped, stem discarded
- ½ large yellow onion, sliced
- 1 container mushrooms, sliced
- 8–12 thin slices organic cheese

INSTRUCTIONS

1. Heat the oven to 350° F.
2. Put the hollowed peppers on a parchment lined baking sheet and bake for 10 minutes to soften.
3. Brown the ground beef with salt, pepper, chopped green pepper tops, and onions.
4. When the beef is browned and the peppers and onions are soft, add the liquid aminos and mushrooms and cook until mushrooms are slightly cooked.
5. Put a slice of cheese into the bottom of the peppers, fill with ground beef mixture, and top with another slice of cheese.
6. Cook in the oven until cheese is melted and bubbly, ~10-15 more minutes, checking frequently.
7. If you have leftover cheesesteak mixture, you can bake it in an oven-safe dish with cheese over top.

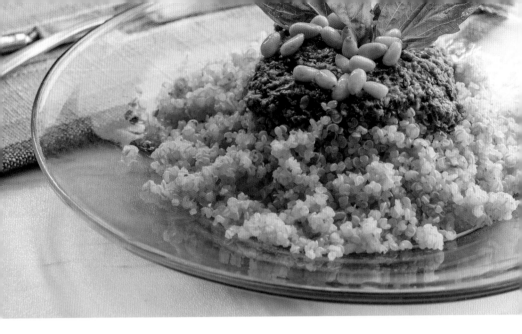

Zesty Lemon Quinoa

| 🍽 **COURSE** Side Dish | 👨‍🍳 **CUISINE** American | 🍴 **4 SERVINGS** | 🕐 **COOK TIME** 20 minutes |

Try this yummy Zesty Lemon Quinoa for a side dish that is both vegan and vegetarian. Your whole family will love this delicious core plan side dish!

INGREDIENTS

- 1 cup quinoa
- ½ cup toasted pine nuts *(or toasted pecans)*
- ¼ cup olive oil, extra virgin
- ¼ cup lemon juice, fresh squeezed
- 2 tsp lemon zest, freshly grated, organic
- 1 tsp ground cumin
- ¼ tsp cayenne pepper *(optional)*
- ½ cup flat leaf parsley, chopped
- 1 tsp sea salt & black pepper to taste

INSTRUCTIONS

1. Rinse quinoa in a fine strainer for a few seconds.
2. Transfer to a medium saucepan, add 1 teaspoon sea salt and 1 ¼ cups water.
3. Bring to a boil, cover and reduce to a simmer.
4. Cook until water is completely absorbed, about 18-20 minutes.
5. Transfer quinoa to a medium bowl along with the pine nuts, lemon zest, cumin, cayenne, parsley, and drizzle with lemon juice and olive oil.
6. Season with salt and pepper and stir to combine.
7. Serve warm or at room temperature.

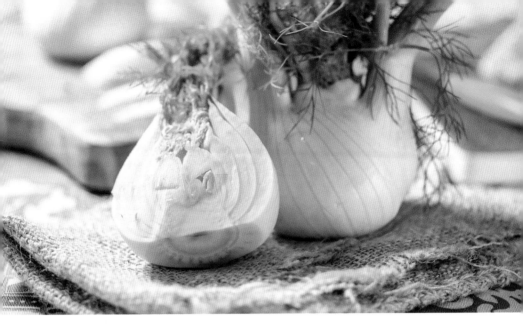

Braised Fennel

 COURSE
Side Dish

 CUISINE
American

 3 SERVINGS

 COOK TIME
12 minutes

This is a vegetable that is often overlooked at the grocery store. It is in the celery family but is much more flavorful and aromatic. When sautéed or braised, it tastes delicate and delicious.

INGREDIENTS

- 1 head fennel
- 2 tbsp butter, grass-fed
- 1 clove garlic, minced or pressed
- salt and pepper *(to taste)*

INSTRUCTIONS

1. Cut fennel in half longways and slice into crescents about ¼ inch thick.
2. You can save the small green tops to garnish if desired.
3. Heat butter in skillet but do not brown.
4. Add fennel, garlic, salt and pepper.
5. Saute until softened. Serve immediately.

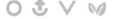

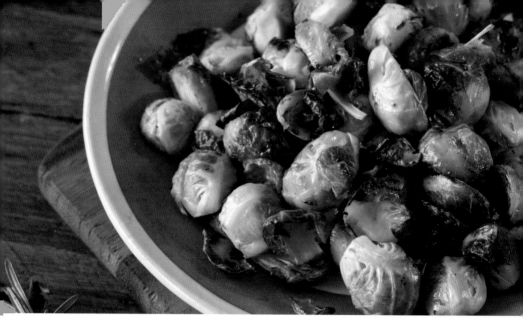

Delicate Brussels Sprouts Sautée

 COURSE
Side Dish

 CUISINE
American

 3 SERVINGS

 COOK TIME
15 minutes

Brussel Sprouts are rich in Vitamin K, Vitamin C, and high in fiber, among many other essential vitamins and minerals. Even the pickiest eater will love these tender sautéed brussel sprouts! With Brussel Sprouts and delicious herbs, this recipe is a nutritious winner at any meal.

INGREDIENTS

- 1 lb brussels sprouts, chopped or halved
- ½ vidalia onion, shredded or finely chopped
- ⅛ tsp dried oregano
- ⅛ tsp dried thyme
- ⅛ tsp dried sage
- 2 tbsp coconut oil *(or butter if not vegan)*
- Sea salt *(to taste)*
- Pepper *(to taste)*

INSTRUCTIONS

1. Heat the oil/butter in a non-toxic pan.
2. Add onions and cook 1-2 minutes.
3. Add Brussels sprouts and spices and saute until crisp-tender (cut in ½ to check).
4. Serve and add salt/pepper to taste.

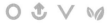

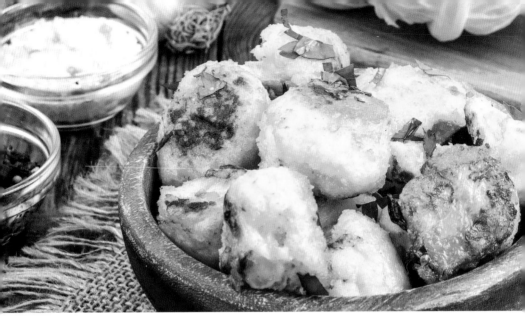

Blasted Cauliflower

 COURSE
Side Dish

 CUISINE
American

 4 SERVINGS

 COOK TIME
20 minutes

Cauliflower with nutritional yeast and garlic is both tasty and loaded with nutrients. Plus, this cauliflower is infused with olive oil so it adds healthy fats your body needs to absorb the nutrients.

INGREDIENTS

- 1 head cauliflower
- ⅛ cup olive oil, extra virgin
- ½ tsp granulated garlic
- ¼ tsp sea salt
- ½ cup nutritional yeast (NOT brewers yeast)
- ¼ tsp black pepper
- ¼ tsp crushed red pepper (optional)
- Sprinkle of cayenne pepper (optional)

INSTRUCTIONS

1. Preheat oven to 400° F.
2. Wash and clean the cauliflower.
3. Cut off and discard the stems. Cut the cauliflower florets into small pieces.
4. In a separate large bowl, combine the olive oil, garlic, salt and nutritional yeast.
5. Add the cauliflower pieces to the seasoned oil and thoroughly coat each piece.
6. Place cauliflower pieces onto a baking sheet lined with parchment paper, or silicone baking liner.
7. Bake for one hour, turning every 15 minutes during cooking. You will want them to look browned.

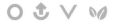

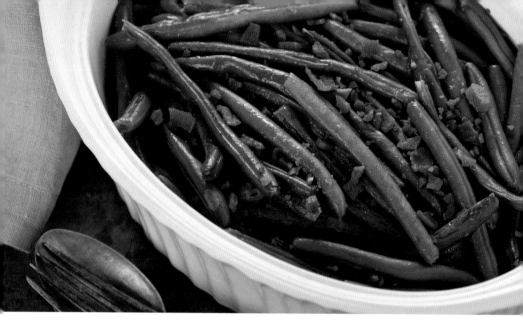

Green Beans with Crushed Walnuts

 COURSE
Side Dish

 CUISINE
American

 4 SERVINGS

 COOK TIME
10 minutes

This super fast, super easy veggie dish has an ingredient that will have people wondering...mmm what is that?

INGREDIENTS

- 2 cup green beans, fresh or frozen
- ½ cup crushed walnuts
- ½ tsp fresh grated nutmeg *(see hint below)*
- 2 tbsp butter

INSTRUCTIONS

1. Melt butter in a non-toxic pan (no aluminum or teflon).
2. Add beans, walnuts and nutmeg.
3. Saute until desired doneness.

NUTMEG HINT: *Keep whole nutmeg in your freezer and use a microplane to grate it fresh for recipes. The taste is amazing and the nutmeg will last virtually forever in the freezer.*

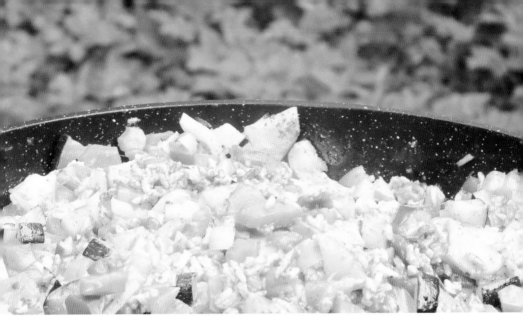

Chile-Zucchini Mash

 COURSE
Side Dish

 CUISINE
Tex-Mex

 3 SERVINGS

 COOK TIME
10 minutes

This is a great zucchini recipe with a southwestern taste. It is super easy to make and can be on the table in about 10 minutes.

INGREDIENTS

- 1 tbsp coconut oil
- 2-3 organic zucchini, halved lengthwise, then sliced
- ½ onion, grated or finely chopped
- 1 can green chiles 4 oz diced, drained
- ¼ tsp sea salt
- ⅛ tsp fresh ground pepper
- 1 dash cumin
- ½ cup organic cheddar cheese

INSTRUCTIONS

1. Heat oil in a large skillet then add zucchini and onion.
2. Cook until soft and slightly browned (about 10 min).
3. Stir in chiles, salt, pepper, and cumin.
4. Mash everything with a potato masher until chunky, then stir in cheese.
5. Scoop and serve.

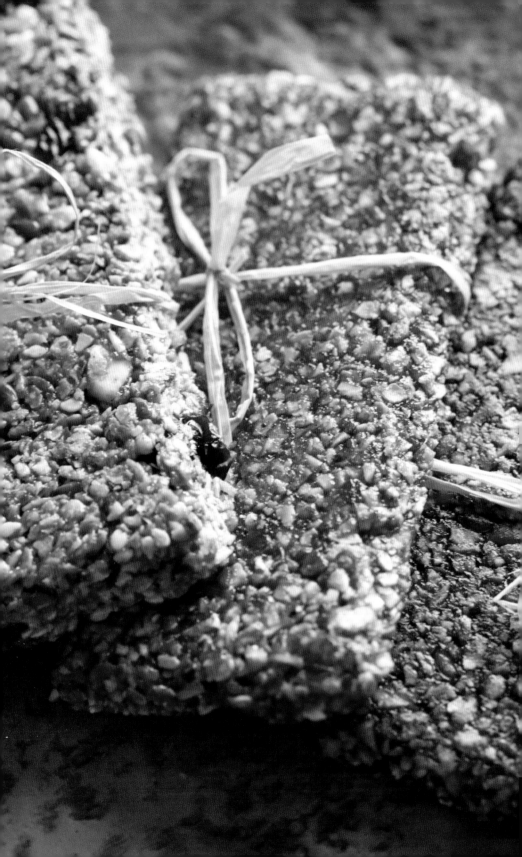

Optimal Energy Bar

Fuel your body with healthy energy gained from MaxLiving Chocolate Grass-fed Whey Protein, dates, low-sugar berries, and chia seeds. This easy-to-make, homemade energy bar is great for breakfast, before or after a workout, or an on-the-go snack. Finally, great-tasting, healthy fuel and protein for your body.

 COURSE
Side Dish

 CUISINE
American

 4 SERVINGS

COOK TIME
20 minutes

INGREDIENTS

- 1 cup almonds, soaked in filtered water overnight
- ¼ cup cocoa nibs
- ¼ cup shredded coconut, unsweetened
- ¼ cup hemp seeds
- 1 scoop MaxLiving Chocolate Grass-fed Whey Protein *(or 3 tablespoons cacao powder)*
- 7-8 dates soaked for at least 30 minutes, and pitted

- ¼ cup goji berries
- ¼ cup dried, unsweetened blueberries
- ¼ cup dried, unsweetened cranberries
- soaked walnuts
- chia seeds

INSTRUCTIONS

1. Using a food processor, mix almonds until it reaches a mealy texture.
2. Add all other ingredients except the dates and mix well.
3. While the motor is running, drop in one date at a time until the mixture starts to form a ball.
4. You may have to scrape the sides and move the mixture around a bit to be sure the dates get incorporated.
5. Place a piece of parchment paper on the counter over a damp paper towel (to keep it from moving around on you).
6. Put the mixture on the parchment and press into a square or rectangle with your fingers into an even layer about ¼" thick.
7. You can also cover with another piece of parchment and use a rolling pin.
8. Use a pizza cutter to cut into squares and store in a parchment lined/layered container.
9. Keep in the refrigerator until ready to eat.

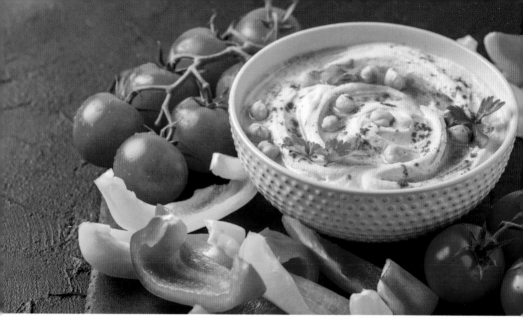

Healthy Hummus
Vegan & Vegetarian

 COURSE
Appetizer

 CUISINE
Mediterranean

 4 SERVINGS

 COOK TIME
5 minutes

This classic hummus recipe is easy to make and very healthy. Serve this smooth and creamy dip with vegetables or try hummus instead of mayonnaise on sprouted grain wraps or sandwiches. With only five ingredients, our hummus dip is simple, yet delicious. Experiment with this basic hummus recipe—you can add your favorite spices like cumin and sumac to give it an extra flavorful kick!

INGREDIENTS

- 2 cans rinsed chickpeas *(~15 oz)*
- 3 cloves garlic
- 3 tbsp olive oil
- 2 tbsp lemon juice
- ½ tsp sea salt *(to taste)*
- 1 tsp cayenne pepper *(for spicy hummus)*
- 1 tsp paprika *(for mild hummus)*

INSTRUCTIONS

1. Place all hummus ingredients in a food processor or blender and mix until smooth.
2. Taste and adjust seasoning if needed.

Desserts

Advanced Plan No Bake Cheesecake
Healthy Strawberry Parfait
Strawberry Cheesecake Fat Bombs
Strawberry Gelato
Mason Jar Berry Cobblers
Chocolate Chip Cookie
Cinnabites
Grainless Strawberry Bread
Banana Bread
Protein-Packed Brownies

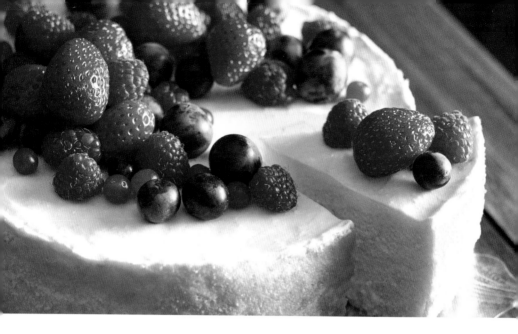

Advanced Plan No Bake Cheesecake

 COURSE
Dessert

 CUISINE
American

 4 SERVINGS

 COOK TIME
15 minutes

Make these yummy Advanced Plan cheesecakes to have a delicious dessert that fits within your diet! Super easy to make and very versatile.

INGREDIENTS

- 4 oz organic cream cheese
- 2 tbsp organic sour cream
- ¼ cup organic heavy whipping cream
- ¼ cup erythritol or monk fruit sweetener
- 1 tbsp grass-fed butter, room temperature
- ½ tsp vanilla extract
- splash of lemon juice

INSTRUCTIONS

1. Mix all ingredients with a hand mixer and spoon (or pipe) into cupcake molds or small ramekins or glasses.
2. Make an optional crust with crushed nuts.
3. Top with fresh berries, boiled berries (for a syrup type topping) or melted stevia-sweetened chocolate.

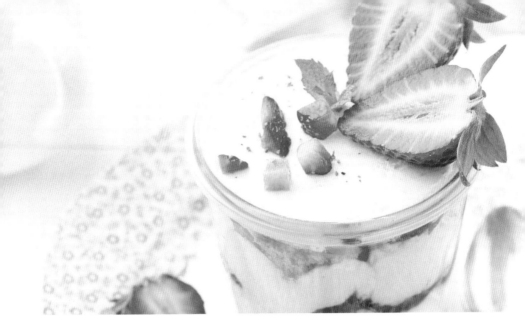

Healthy Strawberry Parfait

 COURSE
Breakfast, Dessert

 CUISINE
American

 1 SERVING

 COOK TIME
5 minutes

This is a favorite treat/dessert. It's great because it is 1) healthy, 2) quick & easy, and 3) the ingredients are on hand.

INGREDIENTS

- 2 tbsp organic almond butter *(or cashew butter)*
- ½ cup organic strawberries sliced *(or any berries)*
- ¾ cup organic coconut milk *(add to cover berries)*
- ¼–½ tbsp "spoonable" stevia *(to taste)*

INSTRUCTIONS

1. Spoon organic almond (or cashew) butter into a cup.
2. Add a handful of sliced strawberries (or any berries really) on top of the berries.
3. Add coconut milk to cover everything, then sprinkle with stevia.

NOTE: *Sweeteners like erythritol or date syrup should be used sparingly on a healthy diet.*

  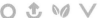

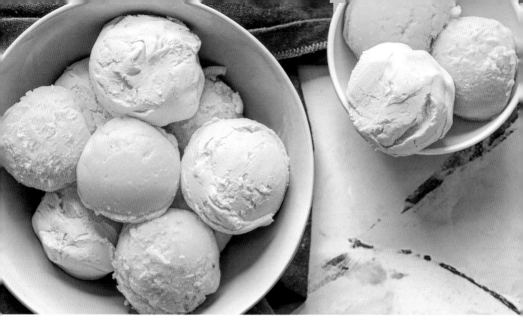

Strawberry Cheesecake Fat Bombs

COURSE Dessert	**CUISINE** American	**6 SERVINGS**	**COOK TIME** 2 hours

This is a great frozen treat made from organic butter and cream cheese. They are a great alternative to ice cream.

INGREDIENTS

- ½ cup organic strawberries preferably fresh
- 8 oz brick organic cream cheese, softened
- ¼ cup organic butter, softened and cut into chunks
- 2 tbsp erythritol *(or 10 drops liquid stevia)*
- 1 tbsp vanilla extract

INSTRUCTIONS

1. The butter and cream cheese should come to room temperature (do not let it melt, they need to be firm).
2. Cut the leaves off of the strawberries and put in a blender with the erythritol and vanilla and mix until smooth.
3. Add the strawberry mixture to the cream cheese and butter and mix with a hand mixer or in a food processor.
4. Spoon into a silicone muffin tray or candy molds.
5. Freeze for 1-2 hours then pop out and store in the freezer.

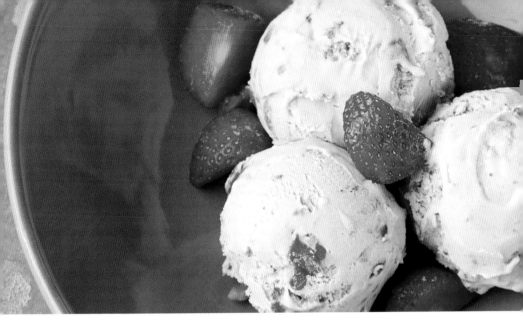

Strawberry Gelato

 COURSE
Dessert

 CUISINE
American

 2 SERVINGS

 COOK TIME
1 hour

A healthy and easily to make sweet treat to enjoy on a hot night. Up the nutritional value of this gelato, while adding yummy chocolate flavor, by adding Max Greens Powder (chocolate) or make this a protein dense treat by adding MaxLiving's Vegan Vanilla Perfect Plant Protein, while keeping the recipe vegan!

INGREDIENTS

- 10 oz frozen strawberries (about 2 cups)
- 1 ripe avocado pit, and peel removed
- stevia to taste

Optional:
- 1 scoop Max Greens Powder (chocolate)
- 1 scoop MaxLiving Perfect Plant Protein (vanilla)

INSTRUCTIONS

1. Put the strawberries and avocado in a heavy duty blender (preferably with a plunger).
2. Make sure you blend it well, then add stevia to taste, (It won't take much stevia because the strawberries are sweet on their own), and any supplemental ingredients, like Max Greens Powder (chocolate) or MaxLiving Perfect Plant Protein (vanilla), and blend well.
3. Freeze until firm (no less than 1 hour), then enjoy!

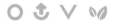

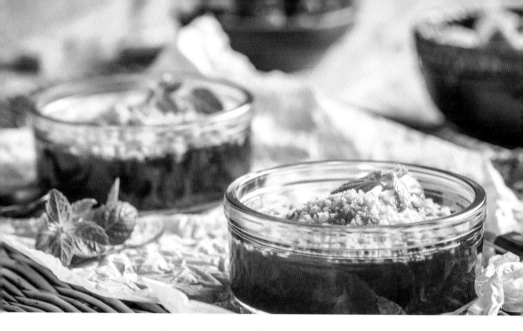

Mason Jar Berry Cobblers
Gluten-Free Dessert Recipe

 COURSE
Dessert

 CUISINE
American

 4 SERVINGS

 COOK TIME
1 hour

There's something about recipes in a jar that make them so much more delicious! Try this easy berry cobbler recipe you can make right in a mason jar. Our gluten-free berry cobbler is perfect to take on-the-go, and they're already perfectly portion controlled. Whether your favorite berries are raspberries, blackberries, blueberries, or maybe all three, customize your mixed berry cobbler to create the perfect fall dessert. If you like this recipe, try our other pie in a jar recipe: Essential Bar Pie in a Jar for a jar pie so nutritious you can eat it for breakfast, and so delicious, you'll want it everyday!

INGREDIENTS

- 3 cups of fresh berries
- ½ cup almond flour
- ½ cup erythritol (like Swerve)
- ¼ teaspoon sea salt
- 4-6 tbsp organic,
  grass-fed butter

Tip: You can also top with cocoa nibs, stevia sweetened whipped cream, or chopped nuts.

INSTRUCTIONS

1. Preheat oven to 350° F.
2. Put the berries into four half-pint canning jars.
3. Combine the almond flour, sweetener, and salt.
4. Whisk it together with a fork and pour it on the fruit, and then top with a generous pat of organic butter.
5. Put the jars in a square baking dish. Bake it at 350° F for one hour.
6. Let the jars cool completely then put the lid on and store in the fridge for up to a week.

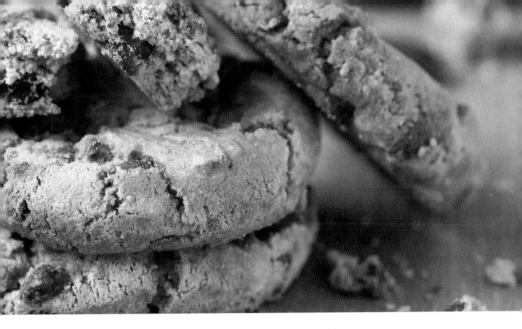

Chocolate Chip Cookie
Gluten-Free Cookies

 COURSE
Dessert

 CUISINE
American

 12 SERVINGS

 COOK TIME
10 minutes

You only need a few ingredients to make these simple—and delicious—gluten-free chocolate chip cookies! Instead of butter and flour, we use almond butter and almond flour in this recipe, making them an ideal choice for those with gluten sensitivities. A healthier alternative to your favorite childhood dessert, try these almond butter chocolate chip cookies next time you're craving something sweet.

INGREDIENTS

- 1 ½ cup almond flour
- 1 cup almond butter
- ¾ cup erythritol (like Swerve brand)
- 1 large organic egg (*or 1 tablespoon flax seeds + 3 tablespoon water/egg*)
- ½ tsp baking powder aluminum-free
- ¼ tsp sea salt
- 1 tsp vanilla extract
- 3 oz stevia sweetened dark chocolate pieces (*like Lily's or Coco Polo*)

INSTRUCTIONS

1. Preheat oven to 350° F.
2. Mix almond flour, almond butter, erythritol, egg, baking powder, and vanilla and stir.
3. Add in chocolate pieces.
4. Drop rounded tablespoons of dough onto a parchment (or silicone baking liner) lined baking sheet.
5. Bake 8–10 minutes.

Note: These can burn quickly, so be sure to keep an eye on them.

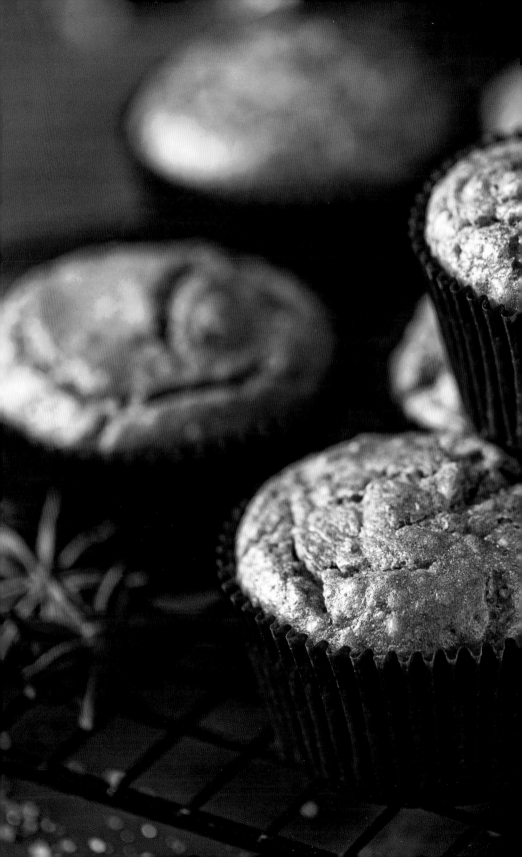

Cinnabites

 COURSE
Breakfast,
Dessert

 CUISINE
American

 36 SERVINGS

 COOK TIME
25 minutes

These were born out of trying to come up with a healthy cinnamon roll recipe, abandoning the "roll" idea and opting for a muffin instead. These hit the mark for sure. You can also frost them with a healthified cream cheese frosting. They are great for breakfast, snack or dessert.

INGREDIENTS

- ½ cup plain amasai *(or organic plain yogurt)*
- ¼ cup erythritol to taste
- 2 organic eggs
- 2 ½ cup almond flour
- ¼ tsp sea salt
- ½ tsp baking soda

Topping:
- 2 tbsp ground cinnamon
- 4 tbsp erythritol to taste
- 2 tbsp organic unsalted butter melted *(or coconut butter)*

Optional Frosting:
- ½ cup organic cream cheese
- stevia to taste
- vanilla to taste
- coconut milk to thin, to taste

INSTRUCTIONS

1. Preheat oven to 310° F.
2. Combine all the wet ingredients into a bowl and blend well with a spoon.
3. Add the dry ingredients to the wet and blend well with a spoon.
4. Blend all the topping ingredients using a fork in a separate bowl.
5. Place cupcake liners in a muffin pan and fill the liners ⅔ with batter.
6. Add small crumble of topping for mini muffins or about a tablespoon of topping for large muffins on top of the batter.
7. Use toothpick or skewer to mix some of the topping into the batter (or just leave it on top).
8. Bake for 20-25 minutes or until a toothpick placed in the center of a muffin comes out clean and the tops are starting to brown.

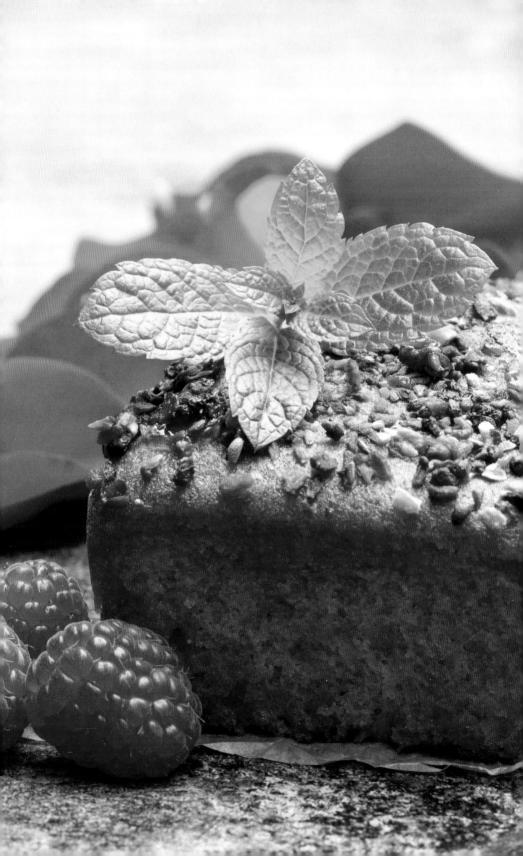

Grainless Strawberry Bread

 COURSE
Dessert

 CUISINE
American

 16 SERVINGS

 COOK TIME
50 minutes

One of the things people often miss when changing their diets are breads, muffins and other sweets. This is an awesome treat that is a great breakfast, desserts or snack. The large slices of strawberries are a burst of flavor. The recipe comes together very easily and can be sliced and frozen if desired. Make them during the holidays as gifts.

INGREDIENTS

- 1 lb fresh organic strawberries sliced (about 2 ⅔ cups)
- dash pure stevia
- 1 ¼ cup date syrup
- 2 cup almond flour
- ½ cup coconut flour
- ½ cup garbanzo bean flour
- 1 tbsp cinnamon
- 1 tsp baking soda
- 1 tsp salt
- 5 organic eggs
- 1 ¼ cup avocado oil or melted coconut oil
- 1 cup chopped nuts *optional*

INSTRUCTIONS

1. Heat oven to 350 degrees. Line two loaf pans with parchment paper.
2. Leave strawberries on the cutting board, sprinkle with pure stevia, and toss to coat well.
3. In a large bowl, mix the flour, sweetener, cinnamon, baking soda and salt.
4. Whisk eggs in another bowl then add in oil and mix well. Add the strawberries and stir.
5. Add the wet mixture to the dry and stir well.
6. Pour batter into the loaf pans, dividing equally.
7. Bake for 45-50 minutes or until a toothpick comes out clean from the center.
8. Cool in pans for about 10 minutes then carefully lift them out using the parchment paper. Use a bread knife to cut into nice clean slices.

Date syrup

1. Cut about ½ pound of Medjool dates into bits and add 2 cups of water.
2. Bring to a simmer over medium heat and cook for about 30 minutes.
3. Let cool for another 30 minutes then puree the mixture using a high powered blender or food processor.
4. If desired, you can strain the mixture with a fine mesh strainer or cheesecloth.

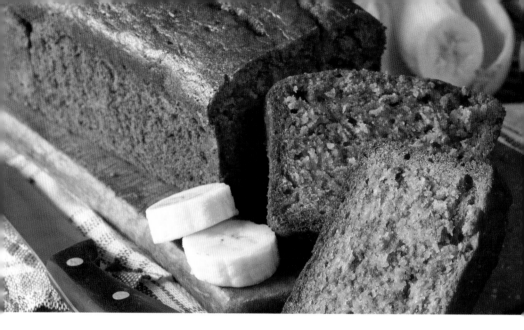

Banana Bread

 COURSE
Dessert

 CUISINE
American

 6-8 SERVINGS

 COOK TIME
1 hour

Banana Bread is an all time favorite but is usually made with refined flours and sugars. This healthier version uses coconut flour, almond flour and natural sweeteners.

INGREDIENTS

- ½ cup coconut flour
- ½ cup almond flour
- ½ tsp baking soda
- ½ tsp cinnamon
- 1 tsp sea salt
- ⅛ tsp pure stevia if desired
- 3 bananas, very ripe
- 1 tbsp vanilla extract
- 8 pitted dates
- 12 free-range organic eggs
- ½ cup coconut oil melted

INSTRUCTIONS

1. In a large bowl, mix flours, baking soda, cinnamon, salt, and stevia (if using) and set aside.
2. Put all of the remaining ingredients, except coconut oil, in a VitaMix and blend on low-med speed until well mixed (do not mix on high speed as it will heat up the mixture).
3. Add the wet mixture to the dry and stir to incorporate.
4. Add coconut oil and mix well.
5. Grease two loaf pans (use stoneware or glass) with coconut oil and dust with coconut flour.
6. Add batter equally between the two loaf pans.
7. Bake at 350° F for about 45-60 minutes or until a toothpick comes out clean.

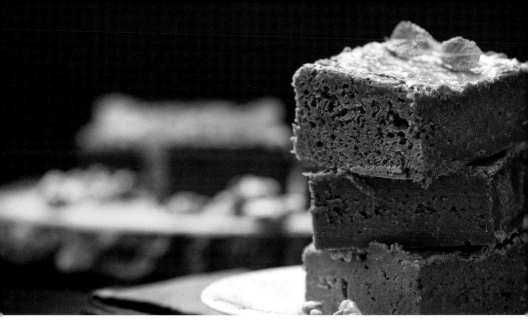

Protein-Packed Brownies

 COURSE
Dessert

 CUISINE
American

 24 SERVINGS

 COOK TIME
40 minutes

This recipe is nothing short of amazing. They taste and look just like traditional brownies but these are actually nutritious and loaded with protein due to the almond butter and whey protein. Make these to share at your next potluck or party.

INGREDIENTS

- 16 oz raw almond butter, smooth, unroasted
- 2 organic eggs
- 1 cup erythritol or stevia to taste
- 1 tbsp vanilla extract
- ½ cup cocoa powder
- ½ scoop Grass-Fed Whey Protein by MaxLiving
- ½ tsp sea salt
- 1 tsp baking soda
- ½ cup coconut milk
- 1 stevia sweetened chocolate bar, chopped

INSTRUCTIONS

1. In a large bowl, blend almond butter until smooth with an electric mixer.
2. Blend in eggs, then sweetener and vanilla.
3. Add in cocoa, salt and baking soda, protein, and coconut milk, then fold in chopped chocolate bar.
4. Line a 9 x 13 glass baking dish with parchment paper and pour batter into dish. It will be thick so you make need to press it into shape.
5. Bake at 325° F for 35-40 minutes or until a toothpick comes out clean.

Appendix:

MaxLiving Resources

Visit our Website: maxliving.com
Order the Align Your Health Book: store.maxliving.com
Order Supplements: maxliving.com
Find a MaxLiving Doctor in your area: maxliving.com/locations

Other Recommended Programs/Resources:

BirthFit: www.birthfit.com
Bradley Natural Childbirth: www.bradleybirth.com
Hypnobirthing: https://us.hypnobirthing.com/
Find A Midwife:
http://mothersnaturally.org/midwives/findAMidwife.php
OR
https://naturalbirthblog.com/find-a-midwife/
Find a Birthing Centers: www.birthcenters.org
Find a Doula/ Labor Coach: www.doulamatch.net
Couple To Couple League: https://ccli.org
Natural Family Planning – The Couple to Couple League: www. ccli.org
Natural Family Planning – The Marquette Method:
www.nfpcoach.com/marquette- method
Perineal Massage: www.mamanatural.com/perineal-massage/
Homemade Weston Price Formula (cows milk) :
https://www.westonaprice.org/health- topics/childrens-health/formula-homemade-baby-formula/
https://www.verywellfamily.com/cord-blood-banking-2633144
Homemade Mt. Capra Formula (goat milk):
http://clubtbyh.com/2018/03/18/mt-capras- homemade-goat-milk-infant-formula/

Informational Vaccine Websites:

National Vaccine Information Center: www.nvic.org
Think twice Global Vaccine Institute: www.thinktwice.com
Vaccine Truth: www.vaccinetruth.com
Mary Tocco: www.childhoodshots.com
List of Vaccine ingredients: www.informedchoice.info/cocktail.html
Children of God for Life: www.cogforlife.org
Dr. Sherri Tenpenney, MD: www.drtenpenney.com

Information on Vaccine State Exemptions:

Vaccine Liberation Organization:
http://www.vaclib.org/pdf/exemption.htm
NVIC: www.909shot.com/Issues/state%20exemptions.htm
Foundation for Health Choice: www.foundationforhealthchoice.com

Recommended Vaccine Movies:

Vaxxed – From Cover Up to Catastrophe
Vaxxed II
The Greater Good

Recommended Vaccine Books:

Vaccines, Autism & Chronic Inflammation: The New Epidemic. By Barbara Loe Fisher.

Immunizations: Are They Really Safe and Effective? By Neil Z. Miller.

A Shot in the Dark. By Harris Coulter & Barbara Loe Fisher.

Adverse Effects of Pertussis and Rubella Vaccines: A Report published by the Institute of Medicine (1991) for the U.S.

Adverse Events Associated with Childhood Vaccines: Evidence Bearing on Causality published by the Institute of Medicine (1994) for the U.S. Congress under the National Childhood Vaccine Injury Act of 1986.

Evidence of Harm: Mercury in Vaccines and the Autism Epidemic: A Medical Controversy. By David Kirby.

Multiple Immunizations and Immune Dysfunction. Published by the Institute of Medicine (2002).

Mother Warriors: A Nation of Parents Healing Autism Against All Odds. By Jenny McCarthy

The Parent's Concise Guide to Childhood Vaccinations: From Newborns to Teens, Practical Medical and Natural Ways to Protect Your Child. By Lauren Feder.

The Vaccine Book: Making the Right Decision for Your Child. By Robert Sears, M.D.

The Virus and the Vaccine: Contaminated Vaccine, Deadly Cancers and Government Neglect. By Debbie Bookchin and Jim Schumacher.

Vaccination, Social Violence, and Criminality: The Medical Assault on the American Brain. By Harris Coulter, Ph.D.

Vaccine A: The Covert Government Experiment That's Killing Our Soldiers. By Gary Matsumoto.

Vaccine Safety Manual. By Neil Z. Miller.

What Your Doctor May Not Tell You About Children's Vaccinations. By Dr. Stephanie Cave.

Vaccine Epidemic: How Corporate Greed, Biased Science, and Coercive Government Threaten Our Human Rights, Our Health, and Our Children. By (i) Louise KuoHabakus, Mary Holland.

References:

1. Schneiderman N, Ironson G, Siegel SD, et al. Stress and Health: Psychological, Behavioral, and Biological Determinants. *Annu Rev Clin Psychol.* 2005;1(1):607-628. doi: 10.1146/annurev.clinpsy.1.102803.144141.

2. Spina bifida. Mayoclinic.org. https://www.mayoclinic.org/diseases-conditions/spina-bifida/symptoms-causes/syc-20377860. Accessed August 22, 2020.

3. Expectant Mothers' Periodontal Health Vital to Health of Her Baby. Perio.org. https://www.perio.org/consumer/AAP_EFP_Pregnancy. Accessed August 22, 2020.

4. Volatile Organic Compounds' Impact on Indoor Air Quality. Epa.gov. https://www.epa.gov/indoor-air-quality-iaq/volatile-organic-compounds-impact-indoor-air-quality#main-content. Accessed August 22, 2020.

5. Smallwood K. Who Invented the Food Pyramid? Todayifoundout.com. http://www.todayifoundout.com/index.php/2013/09/invented-food-pyramid/. Published September 27, 2013. Accessed August 22, 2020.

6. USDA. Choosemyplate.gov. https://www.choosemyplate.gov/. Accessed August 22, 2020.

7. Borggren CL. Pregnancy and chiropractic: a narrative review of the literature. *J Chiropr Med.* 2007;6(2):70-74. doi: 10.1016/j.jcme.2007.04.004.

8. Henderson I. American Medical Association records released in 1987 during trial in U.S. District Court, Northern Illinois, Eastern Division, No. 76C 3777. May 1987.

9. Borggren CL. Pregnancy and chiropractic: a narrative review of the literature. *J Chiropr Med.* 2007;6(2):70-74. doi: 10.1016/j.jcme.2007.04.004.

10. Study rings alarm bell on ultrasound exposure risks. Diagnosticimaging.com. https://www.diagnosticimaging.com/view/study-rings-alarm-bell-ultrasound-exposure-risks. Published August 24, 2006. Accessed August 22, 2020.

11. Newnham JP, Evans SF, Michael CA, Stanley FJ, Landau LI, et al. Effects of frequent ultrasound during pregnancy: a randomized controlled trial. 1993;342(8876):887-91. doi: 10.1016/0140-6736(93)91944-h.

12. Avoid Fetal "Keepsake" Images, Heartbeat Monitors. Fda.gov. https://www.fda.gov/consumers/consumer-updates/avoid-fetal-keepsake-images-heartbeat-monitors. Published December 12, 2014. Accessed August 22, 2020.

13. Fallon J. The Effect of Chiropractic Treatment on Pregnancy and Labour: A Comprehensive Study. Proceedings of the *World Federation of Chiropractic.* 1991:24-31.

14. Vincent A. Benefits of Prenatal Massage. Massagemag.com. https://www.massagemag.com/benefits-of-prenatal-massage-3204/. Published December 3, 2008. Accessed August 22, 2020.

15. Shocking: Why Are Doctors Recommending This Toxic Drink? Foodbabe.com. https://foodbabe.com/shocking-why-are-doctors-recommending-this-toxic-drink/. Updated December 6, 2017. Accessed August 22, 2020.

16. Wells K. Glucola Pregnancy Glucose Test: What I Do. Wellnessmama.com. https://wellnessmama.com/77012/pregnancy-glucose-test/. Updated May 19, 2020. Accessed August 22, 2020.

17. Wickham S. Homebirth: What Are the Issues? Midwiferytoday.com. https://midwiferytoday.com/mt-articles/homebirth-what-are-the-issues/. Published 1999. Accessed August 22, 2020.

18. American Public Health Association Position Paper 8209: Guidelines for Licensing and regulating Birth Centers. APHA Public Policy Statements, 1948 to present, cumulative. *Am J Public Health.* 2002;92(3).

19. Enkin M, Keirse M, Neilson J, Crowther C, Duley L, Hodnett E, Hofmeyr J. *Guide to Effective Care in Pregnancy and Childbirth.* Oxford, UK: Oxford University Press; 2000.

20. Homebirth Study One-page Fact Sheet. Mana.org. https://mana.org/healthcare-policy/homebirth-study-fact-sheet. Accessed August 22, 2020.

21. Planned Home Birth with Skilled Midwives is Safe for Low-Risk Pregnancies. Mana.org. https://static1.squarespace.com/static/5a9072a696e76f194977717f/t/5e998e349bd36660266c03e5/1587121716963/MANAHBData04-09FactSheet.pdf. Accessed August 22, 2020.

22. Margulies M. Should pregnant women be induced at 39 weeks? Washingtonpost.com. https://www.washingtonpost.com/national/health-science/should-pregnant-women-be-induced-at-39-weeks/2016/06/27/e1bb9d16-27fe-11e6-b989-4e5479715b54_story.html. Published June 27, 2016. Accessed August 22, 2020.

23. Mittendorf R, Williams M, Berkey C, Cotter PF, et al. The Length of Uncomplicated Human Gestation. *Obstetrics & Gynecology.* 1990;1(1):929-932. https://journals.lww.com/greenjournal/Abstract/1990/06000/The_Length_of_Uncomplicated_Human_Gestation.8.aspx. Published June 1990. Accessed August 22, 2020.

24. Bupivacaine Side Effects. Drugs.com. https://www.drugs.com/sfx/bupivacaine-side-effects.html. Updated February 8, 2020. Accessed August 22, 2020.

25. Goodfellow CF, Hull MG, Swaab DF, Dogterom J, Buijs RM, et al. Oxytocin deficiency at delivery with epidural analgesia. *Br J Obstet Gynaecol.* 1983;90(3):214-219. doi: 10.1111/j.1471-0528.1983.tb08611.x.

26. Pistolese RA. The Webster Technique: a chiropractic technique with obstetric implications. *J Manipulative Physiol Ther.* 2002;25(6):E1-9. doi: 10.1067/mmt.2002.126127.

27. Newnham E, McKellar L, Pincombe J. *Towards the Humanisation of Birth.* London, UK: Palgrave Macmillan; 2018.

28. McGuinness M, Norr K, Nacion K, et al. Comparison between different perineal outcomes on tissue healing. *J Nurse Midwifery.* 1991;363(3):192-198. doi: 10.1016/0091-2182(91)90007-c.

29. Ashton-Miller JA, DeLancey JOL, et al. On the Biomechanics of Vaginal Birth and Common Sequelae. *Annu Rev Biomed Eng.* 2009;11(1):163-176. doi: 10.1146/annurev-bioeng-061008-124823.

30. Baker D. Public Reporting of High Cesarean Rates to Begin in July 2020. Jointcommission.org. https://www.jointcommission.org/resources/news-and-multimedia/blogs/leading-hospital-improvement/2019/02/public-reporting-of-high-cesarean-rates-to-begin-in-july-2020/. Published February 6, 2019. Accessed August 22, 2020.

31. Backes Kozhimannil K, Law MR, Virnig BA, et al. Cesarean Delivery Rates Vary Tenfold Among US Hospitals; Reducing Variation May Address Quality and Cost Issues. *Health Aff (Millwood).* 2013;32(3):527-535. doi: 10.1377/hlthaff.2012.1030.

32. How Does a Cesarean Affect the Baby? Vbac.com. https://www.vbac.com/how-does-a-cesarean-affect-the-baby/. Updated April 18, 2016. Accessed August 22, 2020.

33. Doucleff M. Rate of C-Sections is Rising at an 'Alarming' Rate, Report Says. Npr.org. https://www.npr.org/sections/goatsandsoda/2018/10/12/656198429/rate-of-c-sections-is-rising-at-an-alarming-rate. Published October 12, 2018. Accessed August 22, 2020.

34. Iannelli V. Should You Bank Your Baby's Umbilical Cord Blood? Verywellfamily.com. https://www.verywellfamily.com/cord-blood-banking-2633144. Updated February 3, 2020. Accessed August 22, 2020.

35. The World Health Organization's infant feeding recommendation. Who.int. https://www.who.int/nutrition/topics/infantfeeding_recommendation/en/. Accessed August 22, 2020.

36. Crepps J. August is World Breastfeeding Month. Dailyjournalonline.com. https://dailyjournalonline.com/news/local/august-is-world-breastfeeding-month/article_792f24b0-c8c8-11e0-888e-001cc4c002e0.html. Published August 17, 2011. Accessed August 22, 2020.

37. Antidepressants in pregnancy increase risk of miscarriage, study finds. Sciencedaily.com. https://www.sciencedaily.com/releases/2010/05/100531155427.htm. Published June 1, 2010. Accessed August 22, 2020.

38. Yu L. GlaxoSmithKline Enters into Confidential Settlement with 200 Families Who Say Paxil Caused Birth Defects. Cchrint.org. https://www.cchrint.org/2010/06/25/glaxosmithkline-enters-into-confidential-settlement-with-200-families-who-say-paxil-caused-birth-defects/. Published June 25, 2010. Accessed August 22, 2020.

39. Effexor (Venlafaxine) Doubles Risk of Miscarriage in Pregnant Women. Baumhedlundlaw.com. https://www.baumhedlundlaw.com/prescription-drugs/antidepressant-birth-defects/antidepressant-studies/effexor-doubles-risk-of-miscarriage-in-pregnant-women/. Accessed August 22, 2020.

40. Nakhai Pour HR, Broy P, Berard A, et al. Use of antidepressants during pregnancy and the risk of spontaneous abortion. *CMAJ*. 2010;182(10):1-7. doi: 10.1503/cmaj.091208.

41. Jury rules GSK must pay $2.5 million in Paxil case re Liam Kilker. Tapatalk.com. https://www.tapatalk.com/groups/ukssrisupport/jury-rules-gsk-must-pay-usd2-5-million-in-paxil-ca-t4673.html. Published October 13, 2009. Accessed August 22, 2020.

42. Vaccines Did Not Save Us – 2 Centuries of Official Statistics. Childhealthsafety.wordpress.com. https://childhealthsafety.wordpress.com/graphs/. Published February, 2009. Updated October, 2010. Accessed August 22, 2020.

43. Livingston B. Vaccinated children more susceptible to disease, learning disabilities than unvaccinated. Personalliberty.com. https://personalliberty.com/vaccinated-children-susceptible-disease-learning-disabilities-unvaccinated/. Published October 14, 2017. Accessed August 22, 2020.

44. Elizabeth E. Toxic vaccine ingredients: The devil is in the details. Healthnutnews.com. https://www.healthnutnews.com/toxic-vaccine-ingredients-the-devil-is-in-the-details/. Published March 6, 2018. Accessed August 22, 2020.

45. Pond M. Vaccine Ingredients – A Comprehensive Guide. Vaxtruth.org. http://vaxtruth.org/2011/08/vaccine-ingredients/. Published August 15, 2011. Accessed August 22, 2020.

46. Taylor G. Examining RFK Jr.'s claim that the CDC "Owns over 20 vaccine patents." Greenmedinfo.com. https://www.greenmedinfo.com/blog/examining-rfk-jrs-claim-cdc-owns-over-20-vaccine-patents. Published January 17, 2017. Accessed August 22, 2020.

47. Vaccine Policy Makers and Conflicts of Interest. Visionlaunch.com. http://visionlaunch.com/vaccine-policy-makers-and-conflicts-of-interest/. Published February 8, 2016. Accessed August 22, 2020.

48. Lewit, K. *Manuelle Medizin im Rahmen der medizinischen Rehabilitation*. Munchen, Germany: Urban & Schwarzenberg; 1987.

49. Gutman G. Blocked Atlantal Nerve Syndrome in Infants and Small Children. *Manuelle Medizin*, Springer- Verlag. 1987.

50. Frymann V. Relation of disburbances of craniosacral mechanisms to symptomatology of the newborn: study of 1,250 infants. *J Am Osteopath Assoc.* 1966;65(10):1059-1075.

51. Towbin A. Latent spinal cord and brain stem injury in newborn infants. *Dev Med Child Neurol.* 1969;11(1):54-68. doi: 10.1111/j.1469-8749.1969.tb01395.x.

52. Miller J. Costs of Routine Care for Infant Colic in the UK and Costs of Chiropractic Manual Therapy as a Management Strategy Alongside a RCT for this Condition. *J Clin Chiropr Pediatr.* 2013;14(1):1063-1069.

53. Fysh P. Otitis Media: "The Miracle Cure." Dynamicchiropractic.com. https://www.dynamicchiropractic.com/mpacms/dc/article.php?id=43069. Published January 31, 1992. Accessed August 22, 2020.

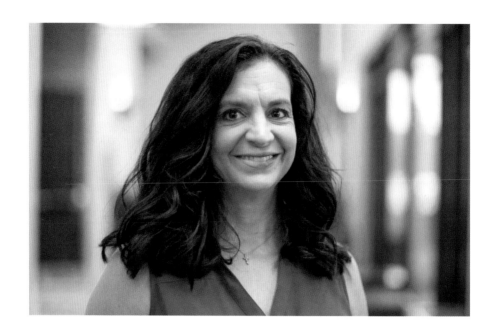

About the Author

Kimberly Roberto is a Certified Holistic Nutritionist and with her husband Dr. Fred Roberto, has owned and operated West Cobb Chiropractic in Atlanta, Georgia for over 20 years. She is a Health & Wellness Coach, utilizing the power of "MaxLiving's 5 Essentials" to encourage people to naturally reach their God-given potential. Kimberly discovered she had a love for cooking at a young age, which turned into a passion for nutrition while in college. She co-authored a book with Dr. B.J. Hardick in 2009 called "Maximized Living Nutrition Plans" which sold over 10,000 copies. Kimberly is a nutrition consultant and maintains a cooking/recipe blog at www.eatsmartmeals.com.

Kimberly and her husband Dr. Fred are the parents of three children, and are passionate about helping expectant parents and newborns by educating them with the knowledge gained through years of their own personal experience.